Praise for *A Guide to Medical Cannabis*

"The right to use and cultivate cannabis should be supported and protected. Chances are you or someone you care about could benefit from cannabis for managing a condition. *A Guide to Medical Cannabis* offers an in-depth look at the plant's medicinal benefits and addresses many common questions about marijuana."

Ed Rosenthal, cultivation expert, author and advocate

"This amazing book meaningfully tells you everything you need to know about cannabis and how to use it to achieve homeostasis in many different ways. I have never seen such a well-written and thoughtfully put together book on cannabis, our human connection to the plant and its history. All humans experience pain in their lives, and reading this book it becomes clear that cannabis can help almost all of us in so many wonderful ways. Thank you for writing this, our community needed it!"

Joshua D. Kesselman, founder and CEO, RAW

"*A Guide to Medical Cannabis* neatly accomplishes an almost impossible task: how to explain the legal, botanical and thera-peutic complexities of cannabis—one of Mother Nature's most valuable gifts. It is an excellent guide for beginners, as well as deepening the knowledge of longtime cannabis advocates.

The book is notable for the wide range of research sources it presents, incorporating the first-hand experience of cannabis activists and patient collectives as well as the latest peer-reviewed scientific studies. In *A Guide to Medical Cannabis*, you will find crucial information currently unavailable anywhere else. I have studied cannabis my entire life and still learned new things about the most valuable plant on the planet."

Steve DeAngelo, cannabis activist, educator and entrepreneur; author of *The Cannabis Manifesto* and Founder of Harborside Health Center and Last Prisoner Project

"This insightful book traces the journey of cannabis from ancient origins to modern therapeutic use. A must-read for anyone seeking to understand the plant's biology, medical applications and legal considerations. It offers practical guidance and expert knowledge in an accessible format for all."

JM Balbuena, CMO of Prime Harvest Inc., author of
The Successful Canna-preneur, filmmaker and entrepreneur

"I am a long-time believer of the medical benefits of cannabis. I've seen it with my own eyes and heard so many stories from people of all walks of life about how using cannabis helped to heal and reduce their suffering, sometimes even saving their lives! Please read this book, you may be able to help yourself or, better yet, help your loved ones!"

Tommy Chong, comedian, actor, musician and activist

"Javier and Nicolás have written the book on medical cannabis I've always wanted to read. They expertly weave in personal anecdotes, expert analysis and deep industry expertise to make this book a must for anyone in the cannabis industry or interested in learning more about it."

Jeremy Berke, founder and EIC, Cultivated Media

A Guide to Medical Cannabis

Overcoming Common Problems

A Guide to Medical Cannabis

JAVIER HASSE & NICOLÁS JOSE RODRIGUEZ

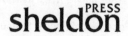

First published in Great Britain by Sheldon Press in 2025
An imprint of John Murray Press

1

This book is for information or educational purposes only and is not intended to act as a substitute for medical advice or treatment. Any person with a condition requiring medical attention should consult a qualified medical practitioner or suitable therapist.

A CIP catalogue record for this title is available from the British Library

Library of Congress Control Number: 2024934081

Trade Paperback ISBN 978 1 399 81559 8
ebook ISBN 978 1 399 81560 4

Typeset by KnowledgeWorks Global Ltd.

Printed and bound in Great Britain by Clays Ltd, Elcograf S.p.A.

John Murray Press policy is to use papers that are natural, renewable and recyclable products and made from wood grown in sustainable forests. The logging and manufacturing processes are expected to conform to the environmental regulations of the country of origin.

John Murray Press
Carmelite House
50 Victoria Embankment
London EC4Y 0DZ

www.sheldonpress.co.uk

The authorised representative in the EEA is Hachette Ireland, 8 Castlecourt Centre, Dublin, D15 XTP3, Ireland (email: info@hbgi.ie)

John Murray Press, part of Hodder & Stoughton Limited
An Hachette UK company

Contents

Nicolás: To Joana Scopel, thank you. From Harlem to Ellery St., with you.

Javier: To my partner, Natalia, and my mother, Liliana, for the never-ending support and push to expand my horizons and always break boundaries.

Acknowledgments

This book would not have been possible without the invaluable contributions of several key individuals. We want to thank Franca Quarneti, for her journalistic rigor, dedication and countless hours listening to transcripts, tuning quotes, and organizing citations that made it possible to complete several chapters. It would not have been possible without her help. Her expertise in cannabis regulation, politics and ecology, enriched the narrative significantly.

We also want to thank Natalia Kesselman and Marian Venini, who dedicated countless hours to reading drafts, identifying overlaps and repetitions, correcting grammar and helping to build a consistent narrative that delivers and clear message. As Executive Editor and Editorial Director at El Planteo, respectively, their extensive experience and meticulous eye were instrumental in managing the content and offering insightful edits.

Gia Morón, Founder and CEO of GVM Communications, a public relations, brand strategy, and business development firm, played a crucial role in connecting us with professionals, experts and activists, making her contributions indispensable. Her efforts in bringing together the right people significantly enriched the content and depth of this book.

We extend our heartfelt thanks to Valeria Salech, whose perspective on cannabis integrative health and advocacy was instrumental. Her dedication to Mamá Cultiva Argentina and her tireless advocacy for health rights inspired us through the challenges of writing. Valeria's passion for the benefits that cannabis provides kept us motivated during long nights and intense discussions. Her unwavering commitment reminded us of the importance of this book, especially considering the patients and caregivers of Mamá Cultiva Argentina, who consistently achieve more with less.

Lastly, we are grateful to Dr. Peter Grinspoon for his inspiring work and kind words. Dr. Grinspoon, a primary physician, educator, and cannabis specialist at Massachusetts General Hospital, as well as an instructor at Harvard Medical School, provided us with invaluable guidance. His honesty, humility, life experience and professional expertise have been a guiding light for us, and his work in the field of cannabis education has been an inspiration.

Thank you for all your support and dedication.

Foreword

Before its criminalization in 1937, cannabis was an accepted medicine in the USA. In the late eighteenth century and the early nineteenth century, more than one hundred scientific papers were written about its therapeutic uses. In the 1850s it was added to the US *Pharmacopoeia*, a dictionary of the effective medications that doctors used. One of the leading voices against criminalization in the 1930s was the American Medical Association. Cannabis was criminalized not for health reasons, but due to racist hysteria and competing commercial interests. In the 1940s it was stripped from the US *Pharmacopoeia*. The Federal Bureau of Narcotics, headed by Harry Anslinger, put tremendous pressure on US physicians to become part of the anti-cannabis hysteria he was creating. Sadly, our nation's physicians willingly complied. One consequence of this acquiescence, along with a tremendous propaganda effort of the US government to demonize cannabis, is that cannabis as a whole, and particularly medicinal cannabis, has been increasingly misunderstood by both healthcare providers and the public at large.

In *A Guide to Medical Cannabis*, Nicolás and Javier provide us with a timely remedy to these decades of misinformation. Their extensive experience provides a comprehensive resource for those seeking evidence-based information on the natural benefits of medicinal cannabis for health and wellness. Their combined expertise in high-level cannabis businesses, research and innovation, policy, advocacy, and entrepreneurship has shaped a book that not only provides scientific insights and practical guidance from experts and caretakers alike, but also explores the socioeconomic, philosophical, and cultural dimensions of cannabis, empowering readers to make informed decisions. This is critical as one cannot fully understand the science of cannabis medicine without also understanding the social context in which this science was conducted.

Nicolás Jose Rodriguez is a policy analyst and journalist with a robust academic background. His diverse career includes international development, policy analysis, and legal cannabis cultivation. His broad experience provides a potent background from which to deliver a critical examination of the power dynamics and regulatory frameworks that historically have governed cannabis. This helps us uncover how societal discourse and institutional control have influenced the industry's evolution. Nicolás's work challenges conventional narratives and seeks to empower individuals and communities by reclaiming agency over cannabis-related knowledge and practices.

Javier Hasse, an award-winning reporter, and editor, has brought unparalleled expertise in the legal cannabis industry from its very inception. As the head of content for Benzinga and CEO of El Planteo, he has been at the forefront of pivotal discussions that have shaped this growing industry. Javier's extensive network of professionals, many of whom were interviewed for this book, and his advocacy for legal access to cannabis have provided him with deep insights into the industry's dynamics. He has interviewed thousands of stakeholders, and has covered a broad scope of issues including environmental impact, economic growth and finance, the latest scientific research and innovation, and the more concrete aspects of the industry by engaging with hundreds of entrepreneurs to understand cannabis from the inside. This extensive coverage and participation make Javier an invaluable contributor to this guide, offering readers a thorough understanding of the ever-shifting cannabis landscape.

Together, Nicolás and Javier bring a unique blend of academic rigor, policy analysis, and hands-on industry experience that makes them the perfect team to author this book. Their comprehensive approach ensures that readers receive a well-rounded perspective on medicinal cannabis, supported by a wealth of knowledge and firsthand insights. In this guide, they cover vital topics such as the use of cannabis for insomnia, neurological disorders, inflammatory bowel disease, as well as for various mental health issues. This is all done with an emphasis on how to use cannabis safely and effectively. This guide stands out as an essential resource for anyone looking to navigate the complexities of cannabis use for health and wellness, informed by two experts who have dedicated their careers to exploring and advocating for the potential of this remarkable plant.

Dr. Peter Grinspoon is a primary care physician, educator, and cannabis specialist at Massachusetts General Hospital; an instructor at Harvard Medical School; and a certified health and wellness coach. He is the author of *Seeing Through the Smoke: A Cannabis Specialist Untangles the Truth About Marijuana* (Prometheus Books, 2023), as well as the groundbreaking memoir *Free Refills: A Doctor Confronts His Addiction*. He is a board member of the advocacy group Doctors for Cannabis Regulation. He is also a TEDx speaker and commonly lectures on the topics of cannabis, psychedelics, addiction, opioids, and physician health.

Introduction

Lately, everybody is talking about cannabis, but there are many ways to approach the cannabis plant: commercially, professionally, out of curiosity, or for cultural reasons.

For us, the women caregivers of Mamá Cultiva Argentina, our approach to cannabis as a medicine stemmed from necessity.

Mamá Cultiva Argentina (MCA) is a non-profit organization established by caregivers who faced the limitations of traditional medicine. We advocate for the legal cultivation and therapeutic use of cannabis, providing education, support, and resources.

Our journey began with a long clinical pilgrimage, moving from one consultation to another, searching in vain for solutions to chronic symptoms that conventional medicine either couldn't adequately address or did so with treatments that brought about adverse side effects.

This lack of answers in traditional medicine led us to seek alternatives, and cannabis became that therapeutic option. The process was fraught with obstacles, though: we had to debunk myths and demonstrate the impact of cannabis on the quality of life of our families.

Cannabis became the therapeutic tool we had sought for years, becoming an ally for those of us who provide care.

The ability to cultivate, harvest, and process the plant ourselves empowered us. We became self-reliant, no longer dependent on purchasing power, pharmacies, or even doctors. We trusted our observations, learned from those who resisted prohibition before us, and found autonomy and knowledge, forming networks of support and expertise.

This plant not only improved our well-being, it also changed our relationship with health and illness.

We became architects of our families' wellness, helping those beyond our immediate circles. From elderly neighbors alleviating arthritis symptoms to cancer patients finding comfort in their final days, cannabis proved invaluable.

We studied its history, biochemistry, and relationship with our bodies, shedding prejudices and fears. We moved from passive patients to active advocates, fighting against prohibition with information and education.

We expanded and also began to help people beyond our intimate circles in our neighborhoods: the elderly neighbor who improved her arthritis symptoms and was able to stop using a cane, regaining mobility; the neighbor with cancer who spent his last days without suffering . . . This plant not only helps us live better, it also helps us die better, and that is something invaluable.

Knowledge, like cannabis cuttings, must be shared to be preserved. We had to change lawmakers' minds to make this vision a reality, emphasizing human rights and the economy of caregiving.

This book is another seed, allowing readers to understand this remarkable plant from all angles. It serves as a gateway for those new to cannabis to dismantle myths and fears, and for those already familiar to deepen their knowledge. By understanding its applications and potential, we hope to further the end of prohibition.

The book begins with an exploration of cannabis's ancient origins and modern re-emergence, detailing its biology and key compounds like THC and CBD, and the workings of the endocannabinoid system.

It transitions to addressing the social stigma of cannabis and its medical transformation, illustrating the shift from taboo to therapeutic use. Middle chapters delve into cannabis's therapeutic applications for various conditions, including chronic pain, cancer, neurological disorders, mental health issues, sleep disorders, glaucoma, and inflammatory bowel disease.

Practical guidance on safe usage, legal considerations, and a look into the future of medical cannabis round out the book. Embarking on this journey has transformed us, and we hope it transforms those who read this book.

We encourage self-observation and the improvement of practices, exercising sovereignty over our bodies. This guide synthesizes all the essential knowledge we had to seek out, offering a necessary guide for those starting their journey with this therapeutic tool.

We celebrate and support the publication of this book, seeing it as another step in the global fight for the liberation of this plant, which challenges the medical system and our definition of health, helping a society in need of healing.

Welcome, and let yourself be embraced by this plant, from which we still have much to discover.

By Valeria Salech, Founder of Mamá Cultiva Argentina (MCA)

1
What is cannabis?

Cannabis is a plant found all over the world. Its history intersects with politics, economics, criminal justice, the arts, and, of course, health and medicine. The plant is rich with a variety of compounds—including cannabinoids, terpenes, and flavonoids—that give it a powerful therapeutic potential. These distinct groups of chemical compounds interact with the human body in complex and beneficial ways.

Cannabinoids are the most well-known group of these compounds. A few examples include:

- THC (tetrahydrocannabinol)
- CBN (cannabinol)
- CBG (cannabigerol)
- CBD (cannabidiol)

Cannabinoids are the primary active ingredient in cannabis. They can significantly affect the mind and body, offering relief from pain, aiding in sleep, and potentially improving mental health conditions. These molecules interact with the body's endocannabinoid system (ECS), binding to receptors that influence various physiological processes.

Terpenes are aromatic oils found across the plant kingdom, and contribute to the scent profiles of many herbs, fruits, and, of course, cannabis. A few examples include:

- myrcene
- limonene
- pinene

Common cannabis terpenes not only define the unique aroma of each strain but also modulate its effects. For example, limonene is known for its mood-enhancing properties, while myrcene is reputed for its sedative effects. As such, terpenes can influence the therapeutic benefits of cannabis.

Flavonoids are responsible for the vivid colors in fruits, vegetables, and flowers, including cannabis. A few examples are:

- quercetin
- kaempferol
- cannflavin A

They add another layer of complexity to the medicinal profile of cannabis. With antioxidant and anti-inflammatory properties, flavonoids contribute to the health benefits of cannabis, from reducing oxidative stress to combating inflammation.

The evolution of medicinal cannabis has led to the development of pharmaceuticals and tailored strains, each designed to maximize specific therapeutic outcomes. This specialization mirrors the intricacies of wine production, where the subtle nuances of grapes contribute to a wine's unique profile. Just as winemakers extract the best qualities from grapes to create a variety of wines, cannabis producers isolate and combine these plant compounds to develop both premium experiences and targeted treatments.

However, cannabis goes a step further, offering not just a range of sensory experiences but also tailored medicinal benefits. Together, cannabinoids, terpenes, and flavonoids are metabolites—substances produced through metabolism within the cannabis plant. These molecules play critical roles in the plant's growth, defense, and reproduction, while also offering a range of therapeutic benefits to humans.

The entourage effect

This synergy, often referred to as the "entourage effect," suggests that the medicinal potential of cannabis is most effectively harnessed when these compounds are used together, rather than isolated.

By understanding and manipulating the concentrations of these metabolites, scientists and cultivators can create cannabis products that target particular health issues more effectively, marking a significant advancement in how we approach plant-based medicine.

This sophisticated understanding of the biochemistry of cannabis is the foundation for its growing acceptance and use in modern medical practice, offering hope for those suffering from a wide array of conditions and enhancing the quality of life for patients worldwide.

Is hemp cannabis? Is cannabis hemp?

The distinction between "hemp" and "cannabis" within the *Cannabis* genus (or family) is crucial for understanding their different applications, as well as legal implications and cultural significance.

The distinction is predominantly legal and centers around the concentration of tetrahydrocannabinol (THC), the psychotropic compound in the plant. A psychotropic substance is defined as any chemical agent that affects the central nervous system, influencing brain function and resulting in alterations in perception, mood, consciousness, cognition, or behavior.

Internationally, industrial hemp is generally defined by its low THC content. For instance, the legal threshold in the USA is up to 0.3 percent THC, following the 2018 Farm Bill.

This legal definition, however, doesn't fully encapsulate the plant's therapeutic potential. For example, industrial hemp seeds, cultivated with less than 0.3 percent THC, have been praised for their health benefits due to their content of omega-3 and omega-6 fatty acids, essential for heart health and reducing inflammation.[1] Yet, this categorization raises questions: if consuming hemp benefits someone's health, does it then become medicinal?

The lines blur further with the use of cannabis for both medical and recreational purposes. For instance, a person might be prescribed medical-grade cannabis oil, akin to a pharmaceutical product, but also find similar benefits from brownies purchased for recreational use. What if they enjoy these brownies with their friends and that brings them joy? Is that a medicinal or a recreational use? The social aspect of consuming these products with friends adds another layer of complexity to their classification.

Table 1.1 Key definitions

Cannabis	Plant with greater than 0.3% THC (in most countries, however definitions vary going down to 0.2% in some cases and up to 1% in other countries)
Hemp	Plant with less than 0.3% THC (in most countries, however definitions vary going down to 0.2% in some cases and up to 1% in other countries)
THC	A psychotropic cannabinoid in cannabis
CBD	A non-psychotropic cannabinoid most commonly derived from hemp

Expanding on this ambiguity, consider the claims made about CBD derived from hemp, which include reducing anxiety and potential cancer prevention, despite the lack of conclusive scientific proof for many such claims.

The classification of cannabis use as either medical or recreational further complicates when considering individual experiences and benefits derived from the plant. The broad range of applications, from industrial to therapeutic, challenges the binary notion of cannabis solely as a medical or recreational substance.

The legal distinction: THC concentration and classification

Cannabis, hemp, and hops probably share a common ancestor, which branched off into different groups more than 20 million years ago. Research suggests cannabis developed during the Pleistocene's warmer periods, which lasted from 2.59 million to about 11,700 years ago, aligning with the Paleolithic era. This time also saw the evolution of early humans, *Homo erectus* and *Homo habilis*.

In distinguishing between the varieties of the *Cannabis* genus,[2] morphology and physical characteristics play a crucial role, especially when identifying industrial hemp grown for fiber, hemp cultivated for seeds, and cannabis plants bred for medical dispensaries.

Industrial hemp,[3] utilized primarily for its fiber in the production of textiles, rope, and other materials, typically exhibits a tall, slender growth pattern, often reaching heights of up to 4 meters.

Cannabis plants available in medical dispensaries, meanwhile, are often bred for their therapeutical components and exhibit a bushier, more compact morphology to maximize flower production. These plants are typically shorter and may have more foliage than their industrial hemp counterparts, focusing on bud development which contains the majority of the plant's therapeutical components, such as cannabinoids and terpenes.

This diversity in physical appearance and growth patterns reflects the specific uses each plant type has been cultivated for, ranging from industrial applications to nutritional purposes and medical use, underscoring the versatility of the *Cannabis* family.

From ancient medicine to countercultural symbol: Legislating nature

From being a cornerstone of ancient medicine to a symbol of countercultural rebellion, cannabis has played diverse roles throughout history, intersecting with societal norms, economic interests, and the legal landscape. Yet despite the challenges of prohibition, cannabis has remained resilient, and countercultural movements have maintained an interest in its medicinal benefits and contested widespread myths about it.

Cannabis distinguishes itself from other crops (such as grape, soy, and corn) and pharmaceutical products (for example, ibuprofen), not only because of its versatile applications but through the unique culture that has blossomed around it. The plant has become a symbol of resilience and rebellion, resonating with countercultural movements and individuals seeking alternative lifestyles or medicinal solutions.

Cannabis culture represents more than just a preference for a particular substance; it embodies a diverse community of enthusiasts, patients, artists, and activists who share a common interest in the plant's multifaceted nature.

As cannabis continues to shape our cultural and legal landscapes, it invites us to reconsider our perspectives and policies, heralding a future where we embrace the full spectrum of its possibilities.

A journey of resilience

Cannabis's long history is closely tied to changes in the Earth's weather, including the Ice Ages. As the ice moved, cannabis was forced into small, isolated areas, which may have led to the creation of new types of cannabis plants over time.

The ability of the cannabis plant to adapt facilitated its spread, and today it grows throughout the world. As human society evolved, cannabis was integrated into different agricultural practices and it adapted further to new environments. Distinct genetic lineages, such as *C. sativa* and *C. indica*, emerged from a combination of human cultivation and natural selection.

Furthermore, indirect archeological evidence found in ancient pollen and through genetic studies offers insights into cannabis's evolutionary path, suggesting it originated in the temperate latitudes of Eurasia. This theory is supported by the pioneering work of Russian botanist Nikolai Vavilov, who identified this region as a center of cannabis diversity and observed cannabis as a "weedy camp follower" near human settlements.

In the early Bronze Age (around 3300 to 1200 BCE), cannabis spread across Eurasia, and by the Iron Age (from 1200 to 600 BCE) it had reached Western Asia and Europe. This era marks a pivotal period in human history as societies developed metalworking skills and established trade routes, facilitating the exchange of goods, ideas, and agricultural practices, including cannabis. The presence of cannabis in these ancient cultures underscores its significance as a resource for textiles and potentially medicinal purposes.

Cannabis in the nineteenth and twentieth centuries

By the nineteenth century, cannabis preparations became widely available in England. Pharmacologist Walter Ernest Dixon advocated for smoking cannabis as an immediate relief for depression and exhaustion. His research further underscored its therapeutic utility and pioneered its use in Western medicine.

During this era, cannabis transitioned from a traditional to a pharmaceutical treatment. A variety of cannabis-based medicines, such as Eli Lilly's tincture of American-grown cannabis, and British Drug House's Indian cannabis tincture, was developed and sold in the early 20th century, while modern prescription drugs, such as Sativex and Marinol hit the shelves in the last few years.

In the late nineteenth and early twentieth centuries, physicians such as John Veitch Shoemaker (1899) successfully treated painful conditions with cannabis, despite challenges related to marijuana's reliability and societal stigma.[4,5] An editorial about "Cannabis Indica" in the *Medical and Surgical Reporter* lauded cannabis for its unmatched soporific and anodyne properties, despite its decreased popularity due to fears over its toxic potential—a concern that has proven unfounded.

This period also saw cannabis being included in mainstream pharmacopeias and its recommendation by renowned physicians such as Sir William Osler for conditions such as migraine headaches.

Legislative setbacks and the "War on Drugs"

In the early twentieth century, cannabis prohibition in the USA began to gather steam. Following the Mexican Revolution (1910–1920), increased immigration from Mexico introduced cannabis into American culture. White politicians vilified cannabis as part of a broader anti-immigrant sentiment, associating the plant with Mexican immigrants and labeling it "locoweed" and "marijuana."

In 1913, California amended its Poison Act to outlaw cannabis, building on previous anti-drug legislation that targeted substances such as opium, morphine, and cocaine. By the early 1930s, 29 states had prohibited cannabis, setting the stage for federal action.

Sensationalized media portrayals of cannabis as a dangerous drug fueled the push for federal legislation, particularly through William Randolph Hearst's newspapers and propaganda films such as *Reefer Madness*.[6]

All this fear-mongering culminated in the Marihuana Tax Act of 1937, drafted by Harry J. Anslinger. Anslinger served as the first commissioner of the Federal Bureau of Narcotics and spearheaded the Marihuana Tax Act, which required individuals involved in the cultivation, distribution, and medical use of cannabis to register with the federal government and pay a tax.[7] For nearly everyone, this tax was prohibitively expensive.

The law was ostensibly a revenue measure, but in practice served to discourage the legal use and sale of cannabis through onerous regulations and severe penalties for violations. Physicians and pharmacists faced cumbersome paperwork and fees, alongside the threat of legal repercussions for any missteps in compliance. The legal use of cannabis for medical purposes dramatically decreased. Cannabis was removed from the American pharmacopeia, and research and therapeutic use ceased.

The Act set the stage for the War on Drugs, initiated by President Nixon's Controlled Substances Act of 1970, which classified cannabis as a Schedule I drug. This classification, upheld despite recommendations for decriminalization, escalated under subsequent administrations, particularly Reagan's, intensifying law enforcement and incarceration rates. Despite recent reforms, the enduring legacy of these policies continues to manifest in racial disparities in cannabis-related arrests and incarcerations.

Today, despite shifting attitudes and some state-level reforms, the legacy of prohibition endures[8] through racial disparities[9] in cannabis arrests and incarceration rates despite equal usage across racial groups.[10]

Counterculture movements and cannabis

The modern cannabis narrative is closely intertwined with the counterculture movements of the 1960s and 1970s, which challenged prevailing societal norms and reshaped drug policies. This era marked a significant shift towards alternative lifestyles and ideologies, fueled by opposition to the Cold War, the Vietnam War, racism, inequality, and environmental degradation.

In the early 1970s, communal living became prevalent in Trinity, Humboldt, and Mendocino, counties of Northern California. In *Beyond Counterculture: The Community of Mateel*, anthropologist Jentri Anders discusses cannabis's role as a catalyst for societal and environmental transformation in these regions during the 1975–1990 period.[11]

A variety of alternative economic practices flourished, including free boxes, farmer's markets, craft fairs, rummage sales, bartering, cooperatives, work exchanges, and land partnerships. These initiatives facilitated a transition towards small-scale capitalism, marked by the emergence of private businesses and services, alongside zoning regulations.[12]

But outside of the counterculture, mainstream opinions on cannabis continued to be shaped by the War on Drugs.

The War on Drugs and its impact

The War on Drugs refers to a group of federal government policies that harshly criminalized illegal drug use, production, and distribution and led, in part, to mass incarceration in the USA. The War on Drugs didn't just mirror societal tensions; it amplified them, embedding deep-seated racial and moralistic biases within drug policies that disproportionately burdened marginalized groups, such as African American communities and other minorities, revealing a pattern of systemic inequality embedded within the legal system governing cannabis use and distribution.

Today, despite the growing acceptance of cannabis and increasing evidence of its therapeutic effects, prohibition continues to disproportionately harm BIPOC (Black, Indigenous, and people of color) individuals, as highlighted by Mosher and Akins in their examination of America's drug laws.[13]

Black individuals consistently face disproportionately high arrest rates despite roughly equal cannabis usage rates between Black individuals and white individuals.[14] For example, in 2022 in Virginia, African Americans accounted for nearly 60 percent of marijuana-related cases post-legalization, despite comprising only about 20 percent of the state's population.[15]

These findings echo previous American Civil Liberties Union (ACLU) reports and emphasize systemic racial bias in law enforcement practices.

In Washington D.C., where cannabis is legalized, a staggering 89 percent of marijuana arrests between 2015 and 2019 targeted Black individuals, harrowing evidence of the persistent inequities in the criminal justice system.

Modern resurgence and medical rediscovery: Cannabis legalization

Public opinion on marijuana legalization has evolved significantly over time. In 1969, Gallup's inaugural survey revealed only 12 percent support, contrasting sharply with 94 percent support of the medical use of cannabis in adults in a 2017 Quinnipiac poll.[16]

The push towards cannabis legalization is multifaceted, with a blend of social, economic, and political shifts.[17,18,19] Many factors contribute to the legalization movement, from public health considerations to economic incentives, to social justice concerns, and the quest for more rational, evidence-based drug policies. This convergence suggests a broader societal reevaluation of cannabis, moving beyond stigma towards a more reasoned and compassionate approach to its regulation and use.

As the medical literature on cannabis and cannabinoids expands, and its potential for treating a wide array of conditions—from chronic pain and epilepsy to the side effects of chemotherapy and multiple sclerosis (MS)—is further revealed, this developing body of evidence is playing a crucial role in shifting public opinion and policy.

The debate on legalization, however, extends beyond medical use. It encompasses broader discussions on human rights, the failure of the War on Drugs, and the potential benefits of legalization, such as crime reduction, and economic gains from regulated cannabis markets.

This transition from a punitive approach to a health-oriented perspective reflects a significant shift in how societies perceive drug use and addiction, advocating for policies that prioritize public health and social equity.

In addition to its medicinal and therapeutic applications, cannabis holds significant nutritional value that contributes to addressing broader health and environmental challenges. Hemp seeds are recognized for their rich content of proteins, essential fatty acids, vitamins, and minerals, making them a superfood that can support various aspects of human health, including heart health, inflammation reduction, and immune system enhancement.[20] Hemp's rapid growth cycle, low water requirement,[21] and ability to grow in diverse soil conditions make it an ideal crop for sustainable agriculture practices.[22] Lastly, hemp's capacity for carbon sequestration and its use in biodegradable materials and renewable energy sources underscore its potential to contribute to environmental sustainability efforts.

Conclusion

The exploration of cannabis's rich history, from its origins as a revered ancient herb to its current status at the heart of legal and cultural transformation, underscores a profound journey of resilience, adaptation, and renaissance. This trajectory has not only illuminated the plant's intrinsic value across various domains—medicinal, industrial, and spiritual—but has also reflected the evolving societal perceptions that have shaped its legal and cultural status worldwide.

Cannabis has transitioned from an ancient medicinal remedy to a symbol of counterculture rebellion, and ultimately to a subject of modern scientific inquiry and legalization efforts. This narrative reveals a complex tapestry of cultural, economic, and legal influences that have dictated its acceptance, prohibition, and subsequent revaluation.

Cannabis has emerged as a powerful symbol of change, challenging conventional views on drug use, regulation, and the potential for therapeutic benefits. The distinction between hemp and cannabis, the impact of historical legislation such as the Marihuana Tax Act of 1937, and the countercultural movements that championed cannabis's reevaluation all contribute to the rich historical context that has defined the plant's legacy.

As we stand on the brink of a new era, with increasing global momentum towards cannabis legalization and recognition of its medical and economic potential, it is essential to reflect on the lessons learned from its tumultuous history. This reflection necessitates a balanced consideration of cannabis's potential benefits against the backdrop of historical stigma, regulatory challenges, and the ongoing need for scientific research to fully understand its properties and impacts.

2
Understanding the endocannabinoid system

The endocannabinoid system is an intricate mechanism within our bodies, crucial for maintaining homeostasis (a balanced and stable environment) and overall health. It is composed of receptors that respond specifically to cannabinoids: either phytocannabinoids, from the cannabis plant, or endocannabinoids, produced in our bodies using fatty acids. Both share a similar structure that allows them to interact with the ECS's cannabinoid receptors, known as CB1 and CB2.

CB1 receptors are found mainly in the central nervous system. CB2 receptors are found mostly in the periphery and the liver, the spleen, the GI tract, and most importantly in immune cells. CB2 receptors in the central nervous system are located mainly in the hippocampus, an area of the brain.

A receptor can be thought of as a lock on a cell's surface, where specific keys—in this case, cannabinoids—can fit to unlock various effects in the body, much like how a key unlocks a door to allow entry into a room.

The role of cannabinoids

Cannabinoids are a diverse class of chemical compounds that play an integral role in the functioning of the ECS, acting as keys that unlock the system's receptors to regulate various physiological processes. They interact with the ECS by engaging CB1 and CB2 receptors located in the brain, central nervous system, and immune system.

These interactions between cannabinoids and the ECS influence a wide range of bodily functions, including:

- pain sensation
- mood

- appetite
- immune response

The ECS is composed of CB1 and CB2, along with cannabinoids such as anandamide and 2-AG, and the enzymes responsible for their synthesis and degradation.

This intricate system, complemented by other non-cannabinoid receptors, is crucial for maintaining bodily balance, offering therapeutic potential across a wide range of conditions by restoring equilibrium within the body.

THC (tetrahydrocannabinol), known for its psychotropic properties, and CBD (cannabidiol), celebrated for its therapeutic potential without inducing a high, are the most well-known phytocannabinoids. The cannabis plant synthesizes over 150 other cannabinoids, each with unique effects.

Cannabinoid receptors: The gateways to effect

Imagine receptors as light switches on the walls of your home; just as flipping a switch can turn lights on or off, cannabinoids can "flip" these receptors to trigger or block various bodily responses.

Our body's cannabinoids, primarily anandamide and 2-AG, with the latter being the most abundant, regulate functions such as pain, inflammation, sleep, and appetite, ensuring the smooth operation of bodily processes.

We produce cannabinoids like anandamide and 2-AG to help maintain homeostasis. Because of this, we can interact with similar molecules produced by the cannabis plant, such as THC and CBD, which can supplement cannabinoids our bodies are not producing enough of naturally.

Dr. Paloma Lehfeldt, M.D., MS, a doctor with over ten years of experience in psychiatric research, neuroscience, mental health, and the endocannabinoid system, recently concluded a study on the use of minor cannabinoids in the treatment of generalized anxiety disorder aimed to find therapeutical options beyond the popular CBD.

With an increase in mental health issues during the pandemic, one of her patients discovered that "CBD alone was no longer sufficient." The addition of CBG, dubbed the mother of all cannabinoids, to her treatment "significantly reduced her anxiety symptoms."

Exploring the therapeutic potential of THC and CBD

Two phytocannabinoids, THC and CBD, have exploded in popularity since states started legalizing medical cannabis. They are the most researched phytocannabinoids to date and many studies are still ongoing to determine their therapeutic potential in helping to managing specific ailments.

THC:

- reduces pain
- induces sleep
- reduces anxiety
- reduces nausea
- reduces vomiting

Please note, THC can actually cause anxiety in higher doses. (See Chapter 11 for more on dosing guidelines.)

CBD:

- reduces inflammation
- relieves pain

As mentioned in Chapter 1, these main cannabinoids do not stand alone: in addition to THC and CBD, other cannabinoids such as cannabinol (CBN), CBG, and cannabichromene (CBC), also contribute to the functioning of the ECS. These, often labeled as "minor cannabinoids," though less studied, suggest a wide spectrum of therapeutic possibilities beyond the well-known effects of THC and CBD.

Table 2.1 Effects of specific cannabinoids

Cannabinoid	Potential effects
CBN	sedative
CBG	anti-inflammatory and neuroprotective
CBC	pain relief and anti-inflammatory

ECS and homeostasis

Maintaining bodily equilibrium is a central function of the endo-cannabinoid system. Homeostasis refers to the body's ability to regulate its internal environment to maintain a stable, balanced state despite external changes, through various physiological mechanisms that adjust bodily functions such as temperature, pH levels, and energy intake, ensuring that vital conditions remain within a narrow, optimal range.

In a healthy body, the ECS acts as a master regulator, capable of influencing and controlling other neurotransmitter systems and the immune system. For functions that aren't self-regulating properly, the ECS releases endocannabinoids as messages to adjust those functions.

Unlike other neurotransmitter systems, endocannabinoids are produced as needed. The endocannabinoid system (ECS) is activated in response to inflammation, which is the body's natural reaction to harmful stimuli, characterized by redness, swelling, and pain. The ECS helps manage this response by reducing and controlling inflam-mation to prevent it from causing excessive damage. This is one way the ECS maintains balance and homeostasis in the body.

The lack of homeostasis can lead to disorders and diseases, as the body fails to adjust to stress, external influences, or internal changes, disrupting normal function and health. Common causes of poor homeostasis that the ECS can help address include chronic stress, inflammation, and pain, as well as irregularities in sleep and mood.

Interconnectedness of the ECS with other systems

Remarkably, the cannabis plant targets key areas within the nerv-ous system, including those responsible for:

- thought
- memory
- emotion
- appetite
- sleep
- energy balance
- body temperature regulation

Cannabinoid receptors are also found throughout the cardiovascular, digestive, and genitourinary systems, as well as in the skin and bones, indicating the system's extensive influence on overall health. The endocannabinoid system's signals are interconnected with those of other well-known systems, such as GABA, serotonin, and others involved in managing pain, appetite, and sleep. This interconnectedness enables these systems to mutually influence their functioning.

The intricate workings of the ECS

As previously stated, the ECS is composed of several components that work in synergy, including cannabinoid receptors found throughout the body (CB1 and CB2), endocannabinoids produced by the body itself, and enzymes that synthesize and degrade these endocannabinoids.

Advocating for whole-plant use

Whole-plant, or full-spectrum, products contain all the natural compounds found in cannabis, including various cannabinoids, terpenes, and flavonoids, which, in theory, work together to produce a synergistic effect known as the "entourage effect."

Dr. Genester Wilson-King, a renowned advocate, speaker, clinician, and educator in the fields of cannabis and hormone/wellness therapy, advocates for whole-plant use in her practice:

> "The entire cannabis plant, including other cannabinoids and terpenes like limonene, plays a role in mood enhancement. The synergy between THC, CBD, and terpenes can help with depression and anxiety, although excessive THC might increase anxiety, while CBD is particularly effective for reducing it. Thus, the comprehensive components of the cannabis plant are beneficial in treating various conditions."

This theory suggests that the therapeutic benefits of the entire cannabis plant are greater than the sum of its parts, due to the interaction of these compounds. In contrast, pharmaceutical isolates, such as pharma-grade CBD isolate, are purified forms of a single cannabinoid, typically produced in a laboratory.

These isolates offer specific, targeted effects, but lack the additional compounds found in whole-plant extracts, potentially limiting their therapeutic potential compared to full-spectrum products.

ECS dysfunction and disorders

Insufficient production of endocannabinoids can lead to various health issues, such as migraines, fibromyalgia, and irritable bowel syndrome. Evidence suggests that cannabis can act as an external agent that can supplement these deficiencies.[22]

First proposed by Dr. Ethan Russo, the concept of Clinical Endocannabinoid Deficiency (CECD) is grounded in the idea that such deficiencies, whether due to genetics, trauma, or other factors, may disrupt the ECS's role in maintaining internal homeostasis. In cases of deficiency, THC can substitute for the missing endocannabinoids and help to achieve balance.[23]

The evidence supporting CECD has grown, with research indicating physical signs of ECS dysfunction in several conditions, such as altered endocannabinoid levels in migraine sufferers and other related syndromes. However, while compelling, the existence and clinical implications of CECD continue to be explored and debated within the medical community.

The dual nature of THC should also be kept in mind. While it may offer therapeutic relief for some, for others it induces dysphoric experiences. In contrast, CBD is known for its broad range of benefits, without the psychotropic effects characteristic of THC.

Clinical implications of ECS understanding

When considering the endocannabinoid system, it's best to view the human body as an integrated whole. This holistic approach contrasts sharply with traditional treatments that focus on isolated symptoms, urging a shift towards treating the patient more comprehensively.

Integrative medicine and cannabinoid therapies

For doctors and patients looking to transition to using an integrative medical framework to help treat their health problems, this means developing a more detailed and time-consuming evaluation process, especially in the context of cannabinoid therapies. Because doctors are looking at your body as a whole, rather than as a series of integrated systems (such as your nervous system, circulatory system, musculoskeletal system, etc.), this requires an extensive clinical history and potentially an hour-long consultation. Such a shift allows for a deeper understanding of the patient's condition beyond mere symptoms, aiming for a complete integration and treatment plan.

When considering cannabinoid therapies, you should seek the guidance of a doctor, especially if you have chronic or debilitating conditions or are immunocompromised. The precision in prescribing the correct type, dosage, and administration method of cannabinoids is crucial, as is ensuring the product's quality due to the prevalence of unsafe and unregulated products on the market. Ask your provider for details about your prescription and how to find safe products to avoid the pitfalls of an unregulated market that may exploit your needs with misleading claims.

If you're doing your own research into cannabis therapies, do not trust unfounded claims about its efficacy and make sure the information you find is evidence-based and comes from reliable sources.

Conclusion

The exploration of the endocannabinoid system within this chapter reveals a biological framework critical to maintaining homeostasis and overall health. Cannabinoids, both endogenous and plant-derived, interact with the ECS to influence a wide range of physiological processes.

Moreover, the discussions presented here illuminate the broader functions of the ECS in mood regulation, immune response, and the delicate balance of our internal environment, highlighting its role as a master regulator within the body.

The ongoing research into the ECS, along with the evolving legal status and societal perceptions of cannabis, promises to unlock further possibilities for enhancing well-being and treating disease. In recognizing the ECS's comprehensive influence across the body and its ability to interface with cannabis-derived compounds, we stand on the brink of a new horizon in healthcare, where the integration of cannabinoid science and holistic medical practices can lead to unprecedented advancements in patient care and quality of life.

3
From stigma to science

In this chapter, we explore the multifaceted journey from cannabis demonization to acceptance, driven by evolving attitudes, patient empowerment, and scientific evidence.

The transformation of cannabis in healthcare reflects a broader shift towards holistic, patient-centered care, where individuals actively participate in their well-being, and evidence-based medicine guides treatment decisions.

Social stigma

Prohibition of cannabis in the twentieth century was fueled by xenophobia and racial stereotypes, unfairly associating cannabis with Mexican and minority communities. The consequences were dire, disproportionately affecting marginalized groups and culminating in mass incarceration for non-violent drug offenses.

This was confirmed by an analysis conducted by the American Civil Liberties Union in 2020:[24]

> "Black people are 3.64 times more likely than white people to be arrested for marijuana possession, notwithstanding comparable usage rates. In every single state, Black people were more likely to be arrested for marijuana possession, and in some states, Black people were up to six, eight, or almost ten times more likely to be arrested. In 31 states, racial disparities were larger in 2018 than they were in 2010."

Despite these distortions, modern research has debunked many of the exaggerated claims about cannabis. Today, cannabis is firmly embedded in our culture: from skeptics to connoisseurs and entrepreneurs, everyone has an opinion on cannabis. It's become a pop culture icon, with the cannabis industry booming since its re-legalization kicked off in California in 1996 and Colorado in 2012, generating a staggering 280 jobs per day in the USA in 2022.[25]

But how did this shift occur? How did cannabis go from being "the devil's lettuce," a demonized substance, to one under reconsideration for rescheduling and a driver of multi-million-dollar investments worldwide? There is no single path to cannabis acceptance. It transcends political boundaries, with both red and blue states legalizing it. Some argue it's a matter of economic opportunity, while others believe this change came from individual interactions between cannabis patients and politicians and lawmakers. Why not both?

Another significant contributor to the normalization of cannabis is the scientific community. Scientists and doctors, through rigorous research, have provided evidence for its benefits, risks, and potential. This evolving scientific discourse has played a pivotal role in changing perceptions and ultimately paving the way for a more nuanced understanding of cannabis.

Cannabis acceptance: An uphill battle

For doctors and scientists, driving acceptance of cannabis among their peers—and themselves—is an uphill battle. One notable advocate for cannabis use is Dr. Peter Grinspoon, a Harvard Medical School veteran with a 25-year tenure. His journey from skepticism to advocacy for medical cannabis is emblematic of a broader trend within the medical community.

Dr. Grinspoon's expertise in primary care and medical cannabis has earned him national recognition. His journey is detailed in his memoir, *Free Refills: A Doctor Confronts His Addiction*.[26] Over the past two decades, Dr. Grinspoon has witnessed significant changes in attitudes among healthcare practitioners. Initially, many of Dr. Grinspoon's colleagues viewed cannabis as a passing health trend, similar to omega-three or beta-carotene supplements. But now, those same doctors are referring their patients to him, recognizing the potential benefits of medical cannabis, in evidence of the plasticity of medical knowledge.

According to Dr. Grinspoon, this transformation is grounded in real-world evidence. When medical professionals observe the positive impact of cannabis on patients dealing with chronic pain and other conditions, skepticism wanes. This change in viewpoints is reflected in the fact that 94 percent of Americans now support legal access to medical cannabis—per several surveys, a testament to the power of firsthand experience and evidence.[27]

Changing patient roles and the impact of information

Over the past few decades in the Internet Age, the role of the patient has expanded, giving patients additional power in the doctor–patient relationship and routes to self-advocate when it comes to their health. Many patients have found new, invaluable information online about their condition and support groups that help them through their health journeys. The latter can be lifesaving, especially for marginalized patients whose suffering can be dismissed by doctor after doctor until they find a competent healthcare provider.

Most recently, the COVID-19 pandemic accelerated the shift towards patient empowerment and information-driven healthcare decisions. With an abundance of information sources, individuals were left to discern the truth, evidencing the importance of patient engagement in managing their health.

Escalating healthcare costs

With insurance limitations and soaring copays, many individuals find themselves resorting to crowdfunding for medical expenses. The harsh reality is that not everyone can afford prescribed medications, even with insurance coverage.

The popularity of alternative medicine correlates with rising dissatisfaction with the costs of traditional healthcare. Four in ten say they've cut back on household spending to pay for medical costs.[28] While this disproportionally affects lower-income households, 11 percent of households with an annual income of above $180K also say healthcare is a major financial burden for them and their families. And as for the care itself, 42 percent of Americans do not believe their most recent healthcare experience was worth the bill.[29]

Information accessibility

In the digital age, patients now connect through social media and support groups, sharing experiences and exploring alternative treatments that may diverge from conventional medical recommendations.

The emergence of "citizen scientists" has become a part of this phenomenon, with individuals self-educating and exploring unconventional treatments based on collective anecdotal evidence. Patients are no longer solely reliant on interactions with their physicians; they're informed by their peers and online communities. Patients often share their experiences, including alternative treatments and medications, outside the conventional pharmaceutical and medical establishment.

However, it is important to thoroughly vet your sources, ensuring that all advice is validated by a medical professional.

The new patient role

Physicians are adapting to this new healthcare reality, where patients have opinions and actively participate in their health decisions. The traditional "one size fits all" approach to medicine is being challenged, and patients seek personalized and holistic care options.

Mara Gordon, a renowned cannabis advocate, entrepreneur, and researcher, explains:

> "Doctors are becoming more accustomed to their patients having an opinion and having a say in their healthcare. But the reality is the vast majority of physicians are not scientists. They're like tradesmen. You have this diagnosis, and they open up their virtual book that says, 'This is your diagnosis. So this is what I'm going to give you, this and this is the dosage. And if that doesn't work, then I'm going to give you this, and I'm going to give you that.' And people are kind of tired of that one-size-fits-all approach to medicine."

Changing attitudes towards cannabis

To treat a patient with medical cannabis, the whole doctor–patient role must adapt. Cannabis is complex, and often requires a fair bit of trial and error to find the best strain, best intake method, and best dose for a given individual. Because the endocannabinoid system and the cannabis plant are so under-researched, there are very few set standards within the medical community. This forces providers to treat patients individually and take the time to get to know their unique issues and needs during medical evaluations.

Cannabis complexity

Cannabis presents a unique challenge for the medical community due to its complexity. Unlike traditional medicine, which often relies on single-substance treatments, cannabis comprises multiple compounds, strains, and delivery methods. Cannabis treatments are patient-specific, involving trial and error because of the unique features of each patient's ECS.

Doctors, then, have to shift to a more patient-centered approach. Rather than prescribing standardized treatments, cannabis-based therapies are tailored to their patients' unique needs.

Cannabis is not a one-size-fits-all solution, but a versatile option capable of addressing a wide range of symptoms and conditions in different patients. Dr. Grinspoon explains:

"It doesn't neatly fit within the traditional framework of randomized controlled trials (RCTs) that doctors typically rely on. Unlike single substances with one specific effect, cannabis is a diverse plant with numerous chemical compounds, and different strains can have varying effects on individuals.

For example, when dealing with a patient who has fibromyalgia, cannabis may have multifaceted benefits: it can alleviate pain, modify their perception of pain, reduce anxiety, and improve sleep quality. These holistic effects on a patient's overall health and wellbeing can be challenging to capture in a traditional RCT. As a result, doctors are becoming more open to considering real-world evidence (RWE), which provides insights into how cannabis works in diverse, real-life scenarios. RWE allows for a more inclusive understanding of the range of benefits that cannabis can offer to patients. This gravitation towards RWE in medical practice recognizes the complexity of cannabis and its potential to address multiple aspects of a patient's health, beyond what a simple controlled trial can reveal."

Cannabis and holistic healthcare

Holistic medicine recognizes that true well-being encompasses physical, mental, and spiritual aspects. Dr. Chanda Macias, a cell biologist with expertise in cancer research, sees cannabis as a transformative force in healthcare and a push towards a more holistic model of care.

The transition to an integrative approach involving cannabinoids requires a more comprehensive medical evaluation. Medical professionals like Dr. Sandra Carrillo now take the time to understand patients' overall well-being, addressing lifestyle, diet, stress, and more. This break from traditional methods allows for a more thorough and patient-centered approach to treatment.

Dr. Carrillo also stresses the importance of continued education and government funding for research to produce scientific evidence supporting the use of cannabis in medicine. She highlights the efforts of scientists and doctors worldwide in conducting research, despite the challenges they face without adequate support.

Challenging the stigma

While advocating for caution and scientific rigor, Dr. Macias has witnessed the life-changing impact of cannabis on thousands of patients. She urges its consideration as a healthcare option, emphasizing the importance of a broader and more comprehensive view of health.

"As a scientist, I initially adhered strictly to the scientific method, where everything was meticulously calculated and measured for specific outcomes. However, my journey with cannabis led me to a profound realization. People seek solutions to their healthcare needs, and it's not merely a matter of chemical formulas or rigid quantifiable metrics. Instead, true health is deeply intertwined with an individual's sense of wellbeing, a complex interplay of physical, mental, and spiritual aspects. This holistic approach to wellbeing varies among individuals and is influenced by their environment and mental state. While some may achieve health through diet and exercise, others require attention to their mental and spiritual wellbeing. The cannabis plant has shown promise in addressing these multifaceted aspects of health."

Dr. Macias also addresses the stigma surrounding cannabis, attributing it to misinformation from government campaigns that equated cannabis with other illegal drugs with no known medical benefits and high addiction potential. She highlights the role of opioids in shaping attitudes towards cannabis, emphasizing that no deaths have been directly linked to cannabis overdose, unlike opioids.

Drawing from her patients' experiences, Dr. Macias challenges the stigma, pointing out that cannabis could have saved lives lost to addiction. She notes that the popularity of cannabis is driven by people experiencing its healthcare benefits firsthand, leading to legalization in an increasing number of countries and states around the globe.

Transitioning to integrative medicine with cannabis

Dr. Mikhail Kogan, a prominent figure in integrative geriatrics and cannabis science, grew up in Russia, where cannabis is deeply stigmatized. Now, he is an advocate for its therapeutic potential. He transitioned his approach to medicine, embracing cannabis as a valuable tool, particularly for older adults with various medical conditions. Cannabis has become a fundamental aspect of his practice, often serving as a first- or second-line treatment, helping patients reduce their reliance on medications with negative side effects. He explains:

"I am in the alternative medicine world, and the strict scientific community, frankly, doesn't care about patients' voices. It's becoming more and more acceptable. It doesn't matter what the science shows. If a particular patient makes a choice based on logic that is not completely crazy, most physicians nowadays will accept and support that. There are still pockets, of course, of high resistance, especially in very conservative institutions."

The landscape of healthcare is evolving, where patients bring evidence and visible results that cannabis is working in them, and this information is gaining recognition alongside scientific evidence.

"Cannabis presents an interesting dilemma for the entire medical, industrial, and scientific complex because it's a weed. It means you can grow it rapidly and get products in a matter of a few weeks or months."

Conclusion

The journey from cannabis stigma to acceptance within the healthcare community is marked by evolving attitudes, patient empowerment, and the compelling force of mounting scientific evidence. This transformation reflects a broader shift towards holistic, patient-centered care, where individuals actively engage in their wellbeing, guided by evidence-based medicine.

While progress has been made, challenges and resistance persist, demonstrating the complex nature of integrating cannabis into traditional medical practices. One significant transformation is the changing role of medical professionals.

Real-world evidence and patient experiences are reshaping the views of healthcare practitioners. This transformation is grounded in the recognition that cannabis is not a universal solution but a versatile option capable of addressing diverse symptoms and conditions for different people, with different bodies.

As such, cannabis's complexity challenges traditional medical paradigms. Unlike pharmaceuticals with standardized effects, cannabis comprises various compounds and strains, making it a unique treatment approach. Doctors are now embracing real-world evidence, recognizing the multifaceted benefits of cannabis that extend beyond what controlled trials can capture.

More doctors are advocating for a comprehensive and holistic approach to healthcare, emphasizing that wellbeing encompasses physical, mental, and spiritual aspects. For Dr. Macias, cannabis holds promise in enhancing these facets of health, as the life-changing impact of cannabis on patients cannot be denied, challenging the stigma surrounding it.

The shifting patient role is another critical aspect of this transformation. Patients are no longer passive recipients of medical advice; they actively participate in healthcare decisions. This transition towards patient-centered care acknowledges that individuals are partners in their wellbeing, a departure from the traditional "doctor knows best" approach.

In addition, Mara Gordon highlights the impact of escalating healthcare costs and the rise of the "citizen scientist." Patients are increasingly seeking alternative treatments and sharing experiences through online communities. The COVID-19 pandemic accelerated this shift, emphasizing patient engagement in managing health. Changing attitudes towards cannabis, particularly the reduced stigma associated with CBD, reflect how malleable the medical landscape truly is.

Currently, physicians are adapting to this new healthcare reality. They are recognizing the importance of individualized care and holistic treatment options. However, challenges persist, especially in conservative medical institutions where resistance to alternative approaches remains.

Dr. Mikhail Kogan's experience showcases the transformative impact of cannabis, particularly in older adults with various medical conditions. He emphasizes the potential of cannabis to reduce medication-related deaths and the importance of patient education.

In parallel, Dr. Sandra Carrillo highlights the significance of evidence-based education in reducing cannabis stigma. The patient-specific nature of cannabis treatments and the need for holistic evaluations challenge traditional approaches.

Moreover, continued education and research are essential to support the integration of cannabis into medical practices, and as the evidence base continues to grow, cannabis's role in medicine and wellness is poised for further exploration and integration.

4

Medical cannabis and chronic pain

In this chapter, we explore the role of medical cannabis in alleviating chronic pain, a condition that impacts millions globally, offering an alternative to traditional, often problematic pain medications. We present an overview of the scientific and clinical evidence supporting the efficacy of cannabis in pain management, and explore the interaction between cannabis compounds and the body's endocannabinoid system. Furthermore, we discuss the diverse types of pain that may benefit from cannabis therapy, alongside patient experiences and emerging research.

Acknowledging the complexities, including potential risks and legal considerations, this chapter aims to provide a comprehensive understanding of the potential of medical cannabis in chronic pain treatment, setting the stage for informed discussions among patients, healthcare providers, and policymakers.

What is chronic pain?

Chronic pain is a pervasive and debilitating condition that affects millions of people worldwide. In the USA alone, it is estimated that over 51 million adults suffer from it, with 17 million of them experiencing high-impact chronic pain that significantly affects their quality of life, according to the Centers for Disease Control and Prevention (CDC).[30]

In contrast to acute pain, chronic pain persists for 12 weeks or longer, often outlasting the normal healing process. Though it can result from an initial injury or an ongoing illness, it can also occur without any clear cause. All this can lead to significant physical and emotional suffering, impacting various aspects of a person's life, including their ability to work, engage in social activities, and maintain relationships.

Traditional treatments for chronic pain often involve the use of pharmaceuticals such as opioids, non-steroidal anti-inflammatory drugs (NSAIDs), and antidepressants. While these medications can provide relief for some individuals, they also come with a range of unwanted side effects and potential risks.

Opioids are associated with:

- addiction
- overdose
- withdrawal symptoms
- nausea
- vomiting
- constipation

NSAIDs can lead to:

- gastrointestinal problems
- kidney damage
- an increased risk of heart attacks and strokes

Antidepressants can cause:

- weight gain
- sexual dysfunction
- an increased risk of suicidal thoughts and behaviors

As such, the limitations and risks associated with traditional pain medications have led many patients and healthcare providers to seek alternative treatment options, such as medical cannabis. An increasing volume of data supports its efficacy. Many patients have reported pain relief and improved quality of life with the use of medical marijuana, and ongoing research is exploring its potential as a safer and even more effective option for chronic pain management.

In this chapter, we will delve into the scientific evidence behind medical cannabis and its potential to alleviate chronic pain. We will explore the role of cannabis compounds, such as THC, CBD, and terpenes, in pain relief, as well as the mechanisms through which they interact with the body's endocannabinoid system to modulate pain perception. Additionally, we will review the clinical evidence supporting the use of medical cannabis for chronic pain, including its efficacy in treating different types of pain, such as neuropathic and inflammatory pain.

Furthermore, we will examine the risks and challenges associated with using marijuana for pain management, as well as potential side effects, and legal and ethical considerations. By providing a comprehensive overview of the current understanding and future potential of medical cannabis in managing chronic pain, this chapter aims to inform patients, healthcare providers, and policymakers about the evolving landscape of chronic pain treatment and the role of medical cannabis within it.

Understanding pain mechanisms

Pain is a complex phenomenon that involves both physical and psychological factors. It is a subjective experience that can vary greatly from person to person. It is influenced by various aspects, including genetics, environment, societal, physiological, and psychological factors. It is not just a reflection of nociception, which refers to the signals traveling in the nervous system, but also the perception of the unpleasant experience. This intricacy represents a challenge for scientists and clinicians who have to deal with anatomical, physiological, cognitive, and affective components.

Scientists have come up with at least four ideas to explain why sometimes we feel pain in a different place from where the actual problem is, a phenomenon known as referred pain.

1 Activity within our sympathetic nerves, which are part of our nervous system that handles stress responses among other things.
2 Because of the way nerve endings split and spread out in the body, pain can spread.
3 Nerve signals may be getting mixed up as they converge, or come together, on their way to the brain.
4 Different pain signals add up in the central nervous system, essentially the brain and spinal cord, making us feel more pain.

When it comes to classifying pain, it's all about where it starts. If the pain starts in the skin, it's called superficial somatic pain—like a paper cut. Deep somatic pain comes from deeper structures like ligaments, tendons, bones, or muscles—imagine the ache of a sprained ankle or a broken bone. Lastly, there's visceral pain, which comes from the internal organs. This might be the pain you feel with stomach issues.

As previously stated, pain is a multifaceted experience influenced by physiological, psychological, and spiritual factors. Various psychosocial factors may enhance pain, including anxiety, fear, and stress, while psychological factors can significantly influence the experience of pain.

Cannabis compounds and pain relief

When a bodily function isn't self-regulating properly, the ECS releases chemicals that the body produces naturally, called endocannabinoids. Dr. Donald I. Abrams, an oncologist known for his research in medical cannabis and integrative oncology, explains:

> "We have this system of cannabinoid receptors and endocannabinoids to help us forget pain. When THC and our endocannabinoid complex interact with those receptors, it leads to changes in the cell that ultimately diminish neurotransmitter transmission, probably either decreasing pain directly or decreasing our ability to be troubled by that pain."

A consensus in the scientific literature suggests substantial evidence supporting the efficacy of cannabis or cannabinoids in treating chronic pain. Both THC and CBD play significant roles in this context: THC is known for its psychotropic effects, whereas CBD is celebrated for its non-psychotropic, sedating, and anti-inflammatory properties.

Dr. Abrams reinforces the real-world applicability through his clinical observations with HIV patients:

> "Many patients had pain and said that cannabis helped with their pain, particularly their neuropathic pain from nerve damage, either from the virus or the medication that they were taking."

This statement is echoed by Dr. Wilson-King, who elaborates:

> "The capacity of cannabis to act as an anti-inflammatory agent,

a muscle relaxant, a mood enhancer, a sleep remedy, and a pain reliever all at the same time makes it potentially ideal for those facing these types of health conditions."

Nevertheless, and despite promising anecdotes and some supportive studies indicating that cannabinoids can offer mild to moderate pain relief, akin to codeine, the research field still grapples with inconsistencies. Some investigations compare the pain-relieving effects of cannabinoids to placebos, revealing the complexity of cannabis's efficacy in pain management and the need for further research.

The dialogue between emerging scientific evidence and clinical experiences suggests a cautiously optimistic outlook on the use of cannabis for chronic pain management. The potential roles of the endocannabinoid system and the synergistic effects of cannabis compounds are areas of interest that warrant deeper exploration to fully understand their efficacy and safety. As the field evolves, consulting healthcare professionals remains essential for individuals considering medical marijuana as a part of their pain management strategy.

Clinical evidence supporting cannabis for pain

The clinical evidence supporting the use of medical cannabis for chronic pain is substantial and continues to grow at a steady pace. Numerous clinical studies and trials have demonstrated the effectiveness of this plant in reducing pain and improving the quality of life for patients suffering from chronic pain. A clinical review on "Cannabis and Pain" published in the National Library of Medicine's database reveals the increasing use of cannabis for pain relief, but also acknowledges the need for additional scientific evidence to evaluate its efficacy. The review emphasizes the theoretical rationale for cannabis's usefulness in pain management and the necessity for comprehensive risk-benefit discussions as its use continues to rise.[31]

In a 2014 patient survey, 97 percent of respondents reported using cannabis primarily for chronic pain, with an average pain improvement of 64 percent.[32] This survey also highlighted the safety and effectiveness of cannabis as a medication for chronic pain, emphasizing its non-addictive nature and mild adverse reactions.

Furthermore, Dr. Lehfeldt discusses the integration of cannabis with traditional pharmaceuticals, particularly opiates, stating: "When you combine cannabinoid-based medicine, the cannabis plant, with opiates, you need less of a dose of the opiate to achieve pain relief." According to Dr. Lehfeldt, this integration of cannabis with traditional pharmaceuticals has the potential to reduce the dosage of opiates needed for pain relief.

Types of pain treated with cannabis

Evidence suggests cannabis can be effective in treating different types of pain, including neuropathic pain, inflammatory pain, and cancer-related pain. According to Dr. Andrea Hohmann, a neuroscience professor who has conducted extensive research on pain and cannabis, the plant has proved to be "effective in treating a variety of different types of pain. Neuropathic pain, in particular, has been shown to respond well to cannabis therapy." Yet, different types of pain may respond differently to cannabis treatment, and it is important to understand which types of pain are most likely to benefit from cannabis therapy.

For instance, neuropathic pain is caused by damage to the nervous system and is often described as a burning or shooting pain. In contrast, inflammatory pain is caused by inflammation in the body and can be treated with cannabis due to its anti-inflammatory properties. CBD, in particular, is effective in reducing inflammation and pain associated with conditions such as arthritis.

Cannabis has proven effective in treating cancer-related pain. A study published in the *Journal of Pain and Symptom Management* found that cannabis reduced pain intensity by 34 percent compared to placebo in cancer patients.[33] Cannabis has also been found to be effective in reducing nausea and vomiting associated with chemotherapy. All of this will be further addressed in Chapter 6.

Meanwhile, CBD has been found to be more effective for nerve pain and neuropathic pain, according to Dr. Duclas Charles.

Dysmenorrhea, a painful menstrual condition, can be treated with cannabis, specifically CBDA, due to its ability to inhibit the Cox-2 enzymes, which help mediate pain in endometriosis or dysmenorrhea. Certain cannabis terpenes, like limonene, can enhance this effect by reducing endometrial pain and size.

Studies suggest that cannabinoids can also make pain associated with gut inflammation more tolerable. (For more about cannabis and inflammatory bowel disease see Chapter 10.)

Patient experiences and case studies

Real-world experiences and case studies of chronic pain patients using medical marijuana provide valuable insights into the potential benefits and challenges of cannabis therapy. Millions of adults live with chronic pain and it poses a significant burden on healthcare and productivity; therefore, seeking alternative treatments for pain management, such as medical cannabis, is a beneficial step to improve the quality of healthcare delivery. Studies have shown that more than half of adult participants found medical cannabis to be effective for chronic pain management, aligning with past meta-analyses suggestive of improved pain management with medical cannabis treatment.[12]

By her own account, Dr. Macias has witnessed remarkable recoveries in cancer patients using cannabis, with improvements in weight, nausea suppression, and overall quality of life contributing to their recovery. Similarly, Dr. Sharma, Medical Director of Gastroenterology at Wellington Medical Center in Wellington, Florida, President of Inspire Care Alliance PA, and the author of *Pursuit of Gut Happiness*[34], has observed significant pain relief in patients using CBD, with many swearing by the results.

The perceived effectiveness of medical cannabis among adults with chronic pain has been studied. In a 2023 pilot study, more than half of the participants reported its effectiveness for pain management. The study also highlighted the need for further evaluation of dosage and mode of consumption to better understand the outcomes of medical cannabis use for chronic pain.[35]

However, note that while many patients report significant pain relief and improved quality of life with cannabis therapy, there are also potential risks and side effects to consider. Concerns have been raised about the safety and effectiveness of CBD products, particularly over-the-counter products, due to limited data on their potential adverse side effects.

Consensus recommendations on dosing and administration of medical cannabis to treat chronic pain have been developed by global experts, highlighting the potential considerations for patients experiencing neuropathic, inflammatory, nociplastic, and mixed pain. These recommendations emphasize the need for expert guidance and the importance of carefully titrating the doses to ensure patient comfort and safety.

Risks and challenges in using cannabis for pain

While medical cannabis has gained attention as a potential treatment for chronic pain, the associated risks and challenges should also be considered.

The side effects of using cannabis include:

- dizziness
- nausea
- impaired cognitive function
- risk of dependence

According to Dr. Abrams, highly concentrated CBD tinctures may impact the liver's ability to break down pharmaceuticals, raising concerns about potential drug interactions. Furthermore, Dr. Duclas Charles points out that THC can worsen anxiety, while Dr. Paloma Lehfeldt highlights that individuals with a history of psychosis, bipolar disorder, or addiction issues should be cautious about using cannabis.

Not to be ignored, research has also shown that high-frequency medical cannabis use is associated with worse pain among some individuals with chronic pain. Increased frequency of use was significantly associated with worse pain intensity and interference, as well as worse negative effects. This suggests that the relationship between cannabis use and pain relief is complex, variable, and may not always be beneficial.[36]

A clinical review of cannabis and pain found that while there is a theoretical rationale for the efficacy of cannabis in pain management, the subjective pain relief from marijuana may not always match objective measurements of analgesia. The review also highlighted the need for additional scientific evidence to evaluate the use of cannabis for pain relief.

Furthermore, a recent meta-analysis of clinical trials of cannabis and cannabinoids for pain found modest evidence supporting their use. However, the study also emphasized the need for comprehensive risk-benefit discussions, as the effectiveness of medical marijuana for pain relief may be influenced by various factors, including patient expectations and media attention.

While some evidence suggests that cannabis may relieve pain, it's essential to consider the potential risks and individual variability in response to the plant. Its effects are often person-dependent, and the form and method of consumption may affect how individuals react to it. Therefore, it's important for individuals to discuss their concerns and potential benefits with a healthcare provider before using cannabis for pain management.

Legal and ethical considerations

The employment of medical cannabis as a treatment for chronic pain introduces several legal and ethical issues. Although it has been legalized in numerous states and countries, medical marijuana remains prohibited under US federal law, posing potential obstacles for both patients and healthcare professionals interested in utilizing cannabis-based therapies for managing chronic pain.

Patients often consider the use of medical cannabis for chronic pain management as an alternative to traditional pain management therapies. However, healthcare professionals involved in providing guidance for patients related to medical cannabis are often doing so in the absence of sufficient data on drug interactions, side effect profiles, and dosages.[37]

However, treating chronic pain with medical marijuana offers dual benefits: alleviating pain and impeding the progress of the underlying ailment. This stands in stark contrast to the severe side effects often associated with opioid use, which has dominated the treatment of chronic pain for years. Considering these differences, it's logical that the shift towards cannabis-based extracts and their lab-created alternatives is gaining momentum for managing various chronic pain scenarios.

The use of medical cannabis for chronic pain management also presents unique ethical factors due to its classification as a prohibited drug across much of the world—although this is starting to change in many countries, with the USA considering rescheduling the plant from a Schedule I to a Schedule III narcotic, under the DEA's Controlled Substances Act. Therefore, it is of paramount importance that lawmakers and law enforcement agencies consider whether medical cannabis should be legalized and how it should be regulated.[38]

Future directions in cannabis and pain research

The potential of medical cannabis as a treatment for chronic pain is an area of active research. Future research will help to clarify the therapeutic potential of cannabis and how it can be used most effectively to manage chronic pain. In the meantime, anecdotal evidence seems to support some of its therapeutic properties.

In fact, observational studies and case studies have helped understand the potential benefits of medical cannabis for chronic pain management. However, there is a need for more comprehensive research to evaluate the outcomes among adults initiating medical cannabis, and best practices in dosing in different diseases and different receptors and populations.

Further, a mixed-methods study conducted in Florida found that medical cannabis was effective for pain relief and reducing the use of prescription medicines, but the drug was perceived as too expensive.[39] As such, the lack of standardization of cannabinoid preparations and the limited knowledge about the side effect profile present challenges for healthcare providers. This is why consensus recommendations on dosing and administration of medical cannabis to treat chronic pain are needed.

All in all, utilizing medical cannabis for the management of chronic pain has proven to be effective in controlling pain and inhibiting the progression of the underlying disease. Cannabis derivatives and their synthetic versions are progressively becoming preferred over opioids for treating conditions characterized by chronic pain.

The exploration of medical cannabis as a treatment for chronic pain highlights its significant potential and the pressing need for further research. Current anecdotal evidence and observational studies demonstrate the therapeutic properties of cannabis, particularly in managing chronic pain and reducing dependence on prescription medications. However, the field faces challenges, such as the high cost of cannabis, lack of standardization in cannabinoid preparations, and limited knowledge about side effects.

Comprehensive research and consensus on dosing and administration are essential to integrate cannabis effectively into pain management protocols. Despite these challenges, the shift towards cannabis and its derivatives over traditional opioids marks a pivotal change in treating chronic pain conditions.

As cannabis continues to gain recognition for its medicinal benefits, it holds the promise of transforming chronic pain management, offering a safer alternative to conventional treatments. The journey of medical cannabis is one of resilience and scientific discovery, paving the way for more informed, effective, and compassionate approaches to chronic pain management.

5
Cancer and cannabis

In this chapter we navigate the intersection of cancer care and cannabis therapy, exploring its potential as a complementary treatment. This section delves into the complexities of cancer, its global impact, and conventional treatment drawbacks, setting the stage for cannabis's promising role in symptom management and possibly exerting anti-tumor effects.

We examine the scientific evidence, including patient case studies and expert insights, on using cannabis to mitigate treatment side effects and enhance quality of life. Furthermore, we address the legal and ethical considerations, advocating for informed, patient-centered approaches in integrating cannabis into oncological care.

While conventional treatments for cancer, such as chemotherapy and radiation therapy, have been the standard of care for many years, they often come with significant side effects that can be difficult to manage.

In recent years, there has been growing interest in the use of cannabis as a complementary therapy for cancer patients. This chapter will examine the use of cannabis in managing cancer symptoms and the side effects of treatments for this disease that affect millions of people worldwide.

The big bad C: Back to basics

Cancer is a complex group of diseases characterized by the uncontrolled growth and spread of abnormal cells in the body. It can affect various organs and tissues, leading to a range of symptoms and complications. Globally, cancer is a significant health concern, with millions of people diagnosed each year. According to the World Health Organization (WHO), it is one of the leading causes of morbidity and mortality worldwide, accounting for an estimated 10 million deaths in 2020 alone.[40]

In the USA, cancer is also a major public health issue. For 2024, the American Cancer Society estimated that there would be over 2 million new cancer cases and approximately 611,720 deaths.[41] These numbers spotlight the significant impact of cancer on individuals, families, and healthcare systems.

The prevalence of cancer varies by type, with some of the most common forms including lung, breast, prostate, and colorectal cancer, each presenting unique challenges in terms of diagnosis, treatment, and prognosis. Advances in medical research and technology have led to improvements in cancer detection and treatment options, resulting in better outcomes for many patients, but it might not be enough.

Despite these developments, the fight against cancer continues to be a priority for healthcare professionals, researchers, policymakers, and individuals affected by the disease. Prevention strategies such as lifestyle modifications, early detection through screening programs, and innovative treatment approaches are crucial in reducing the burden of cancer on society.

Introduction to cancer and cannabis

Lately, there has been growing interest in the potential role of medical marijuana in cancer care. Cannabis contains over 100 cannabinoids, with delta-9-tetrahydrocannabinol and cannabidiol (CBD) being the better known. Some studies have suggested that cannabis may have anti-cancer properties; however, more research is needed to fully understand its potential benefits.

This has been a source of motivation for a growing number of physicians who have decided to delve into cannabis medicine. Dr. Chanda Macias, who has been working with the plant for over ten years, explains:

> "When I started my research, there wasn't a lot of information about cannabis effectively treating the symptoms of cancer patients. This engaged me because, as a woman, I wanted to understand more about breast cancer and its devastating impact

on communities—mothers, daughters, sisters. I just wanted to help in some way. Learning about the cannabis plant, I couldn't understand why it wasn't being researched more to aid people, patients, and the community."

As we strive to better understand the complexities of cancer and improve outcomes for patients, ongoing research efforts are essential. Collaborative initiatives between scientists, healthcare providers, advocacy groups, and policymakers play a vital role in advancing our knowledge of cancer biology, developing new therapies, and enhancing patient care. But what role does cannabis play in these efforts?

Cannabis in symptom management

Cancer and its treatments often bring about a wide range of distressing symptoms that significantly impact the quality of life for patients. In the recent past, there has been growing interest in the potential benefits of cannabis in managing these challenging symptoms, for its medicinal properties, particularly in pain relief.

Cancer symptoms that may be treated with cannabis are:

- pain
- chemotherapy-induced nausea and vomiting (CINV)
- loss of appetite
- anxiety and depression
- sleep disturbances

Pain management is a crucial aspect of cancer care, and cannabis has proved to have analgesic properties.

According to Dr. Manuel Guzmán, Professor of Biochemistry and Molecular Biology at the Complutense University of Madrid, member of the Spanish Royal Academy of Pharmacy, and member of the Board of Directors of the International Association for Cannabinoid Medicines:

"It is most conceivable that the therapeutic activity... is due to the THC-induced activation of cannabinoid CB1 receptors located on precise anatomical sites. This includes, for example, inhibition of nausea and vomiting, stimulation of appetite, attenuation of cachexia/energy expenditure, and reduction of pain, in which effects mediated by cannabinoid CB2 receptors could also be involved."[42]

Medical marijuana has been recognized for its antiemetic properties, offering relief from CINV. A systematic review published in the *Cochrane Database of Systematic Reviews* supported the efficacy of cannabis-based medicines in reducing CINV in cancer patients, providing a valuable alternative for managing treatment-related side effects.[43]

Appetite loss is another significant concern among cancer patients, often leading to weight loss and malnutrition.

Dr. Chanda Macias explains how certain types of cannabis have helped patients regain weight, alleviate nausea, improve energy levels, and enhance overall quality of life:

> "I see other things, like their sleeping habits, improve. And not all cannabis strains work the same. But when you see overall what these patients are experiencing, and they're reclaiming their lives and the pain is subsiding in the process, you start to look at them a little bit closer and feel that you are helping in the way that you wished you were empowered to help."

Nonetheless, she also emphasizes the need for further research to better understand how cannabis can positively impact patient outcomes and advocated for increased accessibility to this potential healthcare solution.

Additionally, Dr. Hemant Kumar Bid, faculty member of St. Louis University and the Cleveland School of Cannabis, explains:

> "Cannabis-based medication can reduce anxiety and depression in cancer patients and make them happier to fight the disease. It can reduce nausea and vomiting and help to sleep. Also, patients with metastatic cancer have huge pain, and cannabis can reduce the pain."

Current research on cannabis and cancer

New research has suggested that cannabinoids may have antitumor effects. Such is the case of a study published in the *Journal of the National Cancer Institute,* which found that THC and CBD had anti-tumor effects in animal models of cancer. This data is backed by another investigation published in the journal *Molecular Cancer Therapeutics,* which found that CBD had anti-tumor effects in human breast cancer cells.[44]

However, these findings still need to be taken with a grain of salt. Further research is needed, so it is not recommended that patients discontinue traditional treatments before checking with a healthcare professional.

Studies have shown that the ECS is altered in various types of tumors during cancer, meaning that the levels of endocannabinoids and their receptors are different from those in healthy tissue. This alteration can affect cancer prognosis and disease outcome, as it can influence the growth and spread of cancer cells.[45]

For example, some studies have found that higher levels of endocannabinoids in tumors are associated with a better prognosis, while others have found that lower levels are associated with worse outcomes. Similarly, some studies have found that certain endocannabinoid receptors are overexpressed in cancer cells, while others are underexpressed.[46]

Cannabinoids display anti-cancer effects in several models, by suppressing the proliferation, migration, and/or invasion of cancer cells, as well as tumor angiogenesis.[47]

A recent literature review identified 77 unique case reports describing patients with various types of cancer using cannabis as a treatment. While the data supporting 81 percent of these cases was considered to be weak, two case series have been put forth as examples of the anti-tumor activity of CBD in particular. Clinical responses were described in 92 percent of the solid tumor patients, most of whom were also receiving conventional cancer treatments.[48]

Pain management

As previously stated, cannabis has also been shown to have potential benefits in managing cancer-related pain. A study published in the *Journal of Pain and Symptom Management* found that cancer patients who used medical marijuana reported a significant reduction in pain compared to those who did not use cannabis.[49]

Expert opinions

Dr. Donald Abrams has investigated the clinical benefits of medical cannabis in cancer treatment and believes it can be used as a complementary therapy, along with conventional treatments, to help patients manage symptoms and improve their quality of life:

> "I believe in the strength of the ECS and cannabinoids. They have been known to have a function in maintaining balance inside the human body. And studies have shown that they decrease inflammation in the body."

Meanwhile, Dr. Bid believes that cannabis has many valuable applications in the field of cancer biology:

> "Cannabis can block the cancer cells. It can block the angiogenesis. It can block the metastasis. People undergoing radiotherapy and chemotherapy who are already using medical cannabis might respond better to these treatments. Research indicates that such individuals could be more sensitive to the effects of chemotherapy and radiotherapy. This means that if a full cycle of chemotherapy is typically required, a long-term medical cannabis user might only need two or three cycles. Essentially, this could reduce the number of treatment cycles needed."

Risks and controversies

In the realm of cancer care, the integration of cannabis as a potential therapeutic agent has brought with it both intrigue and skepticism. While its benefits are being increasingly recognized, it is crucial to acknowledge the associated risks and controversies that accompany its use in this context.

As always, stigma plays a role in the inconveniences of prescribing medical marijuana for cancer patients. Such is the experience of Mara Gordon: "When I first started working with this, I had family members who told me that they couldn't believe

I was a drug dealer, especially since I was specializing in pediatric cancer."

As such, clinical trials are essential in evaluating the safety and efficacy of cannabis-based therapies. A study published in the *Journal of Clinical Oncology* found that cannabis use was associated with a higher risk of drug interactions in cancer patients.[50] Therefore, it is crucial to conduct rigorous clinical trials to ensure that cannabis-based therapies do not pose any significant risks to cancer patients.

However, there is also the problem of false hope, which comes with the misguided belief that cannabis is a cure-all. As Dr. Abram says:

> "There is no convincing evidence in human beings that cannabis does anything to inhibit cancer growth. And so, one of the things that used to upset me the most was when patients waited for 4 – 6 months to see me with a treatable or curable malignancy; patients who were treating themselves only with cannabis, thinking that I would say that's a good idea."

But just as it is inaccurate to say that cannabis in itself cures cancer, it is to say that it causes it:

> "Some people are still concerned that cannabis increases the risk of cancer, but this is incorrect. Cannabis may actually decrease the risk of bladder cancer, and possibly lung cancer."

Furthermore, Dr. Bid acknowledges the inherent side effects associated with all forms of medication, including cannabis:

> "Every medicine has side effects, right? So basically, if you search for any medicine into Google, you will see that in modern medicine you will find so many different side effects. Same as cannabis, it also has side effects."

As the potential benefits of medical marijuana in cancer care continue to emerge, it becomes essential to address the complex web of legal and ethical considerations that surround its usage. From varying global legal frameworks to challenging moral dilemmas, navigating this terrain requires careful consideration and thoughtful deliberation.

Legal and ethical considerations

First, the legal status of cannabis differs significantly across the globe. Some nations permit its use for medicinal purposes, whereas others maintain strict prohibitions against it. For instance, Canada and several European Union member states allow medical marijuana use under specific conditions, while countries such as China and Japan strictly ban it. These disparities pose a challenge for cancer patients seeking access to cannabis as part of their treatment plan.

Second, the ethical implications of employing cannabis in cancer therapy demand scrutiny. Patient autonomy, informed consent, and the potential for harm are central themes in this debate.

Healthcare providers must weigh the potential benefits of cannabis against its known harms and side effects while engaging in open dialogue with their patients to discuss the risks and limitations of cannabis use. This way, they can ensure that each individual makes informed decisions based on their circumstances and preferences.

Yet, the guidelines for the use of cannabis in the treatment of cancer and/or the management of its symptoms are still being developed, and to achieve a more comprehensive framework for the plant's medical value, it is important that everyone chips in.

For example, a study conducted by the American Society of Clinical Oncology (ASCO) revealed that nearly half of oncologists surveyed reported having discussed cannabis with their patients, yet less than 5 percent felt adequately prepared to guide its safe and effective use. To bridge this knowledge gap, ASCO developed educational resources aimed at equipping clinicians with the necessary tools to counsel their patients on cannabis use.

Additionally, the National Comprehensive Cancer Network (NCCN), a nonprofit alliance of leading cancer centers dedicated to improving patient outcomes, provides guidelines for healthcare providers on the appropriate use of cannabis in cancer care.[51]

Lastly, the role of public opinion and social acceptance cannot be overlooked. As society continues to struggle with the legalization of adult-use marijuana, healthcare providers may encounter resistance from patients and families who view cannabis solely through the lens of recreation rather than as a legitimate medical intervention. It is key for healthcare providers to educate their communities about the potential benefits and risks of cannabis use in cancer therapy, fostering greater awareness and understanding amongst stakeholders.

By engaging in open dialogues with patients, consulting reputable sources, and staying abreast of emerging trends in cannabis research, healthcare providers can help guide their patients along the path towards optimal wellness and symptom management during their cancer journey.

Through this collaborative effort, the field of cancer care stands to benefit from the promising possibilities offered by cannabis, while simultaneously safeguarding against potential harms and complications.

Future directions and potential therapies

Future research should focus on understanding the mechanisms of action of cannabinoids in cancer cells, identifying specific cannabinoids with anti-cancer properties, and conducting clinical trials to evaluate the safety and efficacy of cannabis-based therapies.

Dr. Paola Massi, a researcher focusing on the pharmacological exploitation of cannabinoids in cancer treatment, explains:

> "Future research should focus on developing new cannabis-based therapies for cancer patients. While more research is needed, the potential for cannabis to be used as a complementary therapy in cancer care is promising."

One area of research that holds significant promise is the identification of specific cannabinoids with anti-cancer properties. For instance, a study published in the *International Journal of Molecular Sciences* found that CBD inhibited the growth of breast cancer cells in vitro.[52]

Moreover, cannabis-based therapies like Sativex (a combination of THC and CBD) and Epidiolex (pure CBD) have been approved for medical use in some countries. These therapies may provide new treatment options for cancer patients in the future. Dr. Abrams notes the potential of cannabis-based therapies:

"There are a lot of different cannabinoids that have different effects. There's a lot of potential for developing new drugs that are based on the different cannabinoids that are in the plant."

Dr. Bid highlights the ongoing research in the field of cancer biology:

"There are so many different clinical trials going on worldwide and globally that we are looking forward to seeing what is next in the field of cancer biology."

As the scientific community continues to explore the potential of medical marijuana in cancer care, it is essential to remain vigilant and continue to research to ensure that cannabis-based therapies are safe and effective for cancer patients.

Conclusion

Upon reflecting on the intricate pathways of cannabis and cancer care, Dr. Bid says, "Cannabis is not a magical drug. It's all about what you are looking for." These words encapsulate the complexities of integrating cannabis into oncology, a journey marked by nuance, hope, and a steadfast commitment to patient-centered care.

It is becoming increasingly clear that while the road ahead may be rocky and uncertain, it is also full of promise and possibility. The current body of research showcases the potential benefits of cannabis as a complementary therapy for managing symptoms and improving the quality of life for cancer patients.

Looking to the future, it is imperative that we continue to tread this path with diligence and, especially, with compassion, and let ourselves be guided by the principles of evidence-based practice, patient advocacy, and unbiased research. Dr. Bid's reminder that "the sooner the diagnosis, the better the prognosis" serves as a poignant call to action—urging us to embrace early intervention and innovation in our quest to enhance outcomes for those battling cancer.

6

Cannabis therapy for neurological disorders

This chapter ventures into the promising realm of cannabis therapy for neurological disorders, offering insights into its potential to manage conditions like epilepsy, multiple sclerosis, and neurodegenerative diseases.

Highlighting expert perspectives and patient experiences, this chapter delves into the complexities of using cannabis as a complementary treatment, exploring its neuroprotective, anti-inflammatory, and analgesic properties, and underscores the importance of ongoing research to fully harness cannabis's therapeutic potential.

Neurological disorders and cannabis

Neurological disorders, encompassing a diverse array of conditions affecting the brain, spinal cord, and nerves, pose significant challenges to millions of individuals worldwide. In a 2007 report, the World Health Organization estimated that neurological disorders affect up to one billion people globally, with 50 million individuals suffering from epilepsy and 24 million from Alzheimer's and other dementias.[53]

Meanwhile, a study released by *The Lancet Neurology* revealed that neurological disorders, ranging from migraine to stroke, Parkinson's disease, and dementia, are now the leading cause of ill health worldwide, causing 11.1 million deaths in 2021 alone.[54] This study emphasized the rising prevalence of neurological disorders, with 43 percent of the world's population—3.4 billion people—affected in 2021, a dramatic increase over the past three decades.

Neurological care is a complex terrain, in which traditional treatment approaches have centered on pharmacological interventions, physical therapy, and surgical procedures aimed at managing symptoms and slowing disease progression. However, a shift is underway with the exploration of cannabis-based therapies as potential adjuncts or alternatives in the management of these challenging conditions.

Dr. Mikhail Kogan, medical director of the George Washington University Center for Integrative Medicine and member of the Board of Advisors at Doctors for Cannabis Regulation (DFCR), emphasizes the critical role of cannabis in conditions such as Alzheimer's, Parkinson's, and multiple sclerosis. This patient population usually sees a decline in endogenous cannabinoid production, suggesting that supplementing with exogenous cannabinoids can lead to significant improvements in symptomatology.

The integration of cannabis into neurological care represents a promising frontier in therapeutic innovation. By leveraging the neuroprotective, anti-inflammatory, and analgesic properties of cannabinoids, healthcare providers have an opportunity to enhance treatment strategies and improve outcomes for individuals grappling with these complex disorders. Hereby, the exploration of cannabis therapy opens new possibilities for personalized and effective interventions that prioritize patient well-being and quality of life.

Cannabis and epilepsy

Epilepsy is a neurological disorder characterized by recurrent seizures, and is a challenging condition to manage effectively. In recent years, the spotlight has turned to cannabis, particularly CBD, as a potential treatment option for epilepsy patients.

One of the most compelling success stories in cannabis treatment for epilepsy is that of Charlotte Figi, a young girl with Dravet syndrome. By the time she turned five years old, she was experiencing up to 300 seizures a week. Her parents, frantic and running out of treatment options, tried giving her a strain with high CBD and low THC. Her seizures dramatically reduced from 300 a week to fewer than ten.[55] This remarkable outcome paved the way for FDA approval of the CBD-based oral solution Epidiolex for Lennox-Gastaut syndrome and Dravet syndrome, marking a significant milestone in epilepsy treatment.

Figi's story continues to resonate deeply within the medical community, even after her untimely passing in 2020 due to complications from COVID-19. Her journey not only brought hope to countless families grappling with epilepsy but also catalyzed crucial research into the therapeutic potential of CBD.

Dr. Monica Werkheiser is a seasoned pharmacist deeply immersed in the medical marijuana field:

> "Each neurological and neurodegenerative disease presents its own set of complexities, demanding a dynamic and individualized approach to treatment. Particularly with epilepsy, where the disease's progression and the patient's response to cannabis can vary widely, it's essential to remain adaptable, tailoring the treatment to the patient's evolving needs."

As such, epilepsy has significantly influenced the medical cannabis movement, especially in pediatric cases, and it serves as a poignant example of the broader challenges faced in the field of neurodegenerative disorders. Dr. Werkheiser noted an interesting paradox: despite the push for medical cannabis sparked by childhood epilepsy cases, adults with epilepsy have become the primary beneficiaries of her practice.

Three critical factors have emerged in the management of epilepsy:

1 the primary goal of seizure control
2 the management of medication side effects
3 the intricate balance between THC and CBD in treatment protocols.

Pressing on the importance of high CBD formulations, Dr. Werkheiser emphasizes their neuroprotective properties, which are paramount in preventing seizures. Yet, the balancing act between THC and CBD is pivotal in addressing the side effects of traditional epilepsy medications. Cannabis can influence the seizure threshold, necessitating a careful adjustment of THC and CBD ratios to mitigate medication side effects while maintaining seizure control.

CBD is a complex compound, and it has more than 46 targets in our body. This complexity evidences the multifaceted nature of CBD's therapeutic effects and its potential to modulate various physiological processes implicated in epilepsy.

In addition, studies have shown that CBD exerts anticonvulsant effects through multiple mechanisms, including modulation of neurotransmitter release, ion channels, and inflammatory pathways in the brain. A systematic review and meta-analysis published in the medical publication *Drugs* analyzed the efficacy and safety of CBD as an adjunctive therapy for refractory epilepsy, reporting a significant reduction in seizure frequency among patients receiving CBD compared to placebo.[56]

The neuroprotective properties of CBD have also garnered attention in epilepsy research, with preclinical studies demonstrating its ability to reduce neuronal damage and inflammation in animal models of seizures.[57] Furthermore, CBD's favorable safety profile and limited side effects make it an attractive option for individuals seeking alternative or complementary approaches to managing their epilepsy.

Cannabis in treating multiple sclerosis

Multiple sclerosis is a chronic autoimmune disease that affects the central nervous system, leading to a range of debilitating symptoms such as:

- muscle spasms and weakness
- fatigue
- impaired coordination
- mobility problems
- pain
- blurry vision or loss of vision
- cognitive problems

The quest for effective treatments to alleviate this complex affliction has led researchers and patients alike to explore the potential benefits of cannabis.

Research has shown that cannabinoids interact with the endocannabinoid system in the body, which plays a crucial role in regulating various physiological processes such as pain perception, inflammation, and immune responses. This interaction has been linked to potential neuroprotective, anti-inflammatory, and analgesic effects that may benefit individuals with MS by modulating disease progression and symptom severity.[58]

One of the significant achievements in the use of cannabis for managing MS symptoms is its impact on spasticity. Clinical trials have demonstrated that cannabinoids can effectively reduce muscle spasticity in patients with MS, leading to improved mobility and quality of life.[59, 60, 61]

Moreover, CBD has emerged as a promising candidate for managing neuropathic pain in individuals with MS. For more information on neuropathic pain and medical cannabis, refer to Chapter 5.

Cannabis and neurodegenerative disorders

In the exploration of medical cannabis for the treatment of neurodegenerative disorders, such as Alzheimer's and Parkinson's diseases, the conversation transcends mere academic interest, entering a realm where empirical evidence and patient experiences intertwine. These conditions, characterized by the progressive degeneration of neurons, present a formidable challenge, yet medical marijuana is proving to be a useful tool for symptom management and potential disease modification.

The National Center for Biotechnology Information (NCBI) has noted that cannabinoids like THC and CBD exhibit neuroprotective, anti-inflammatory, and antioxidant effects. This interaction with the ECS suggests a pathway to combat the mechanisms of neurodegeneration, fostering neuron protection, survival, and neuroplasticity. Clinical studies highlight the reduction of neuroinflammation and improvement in cognitive functions, offering a glimpse into the therapeutic horizon for these debilitating conditions.[62,63]

According to a study published in *Clinical Neuropharmacology*, researchers concluded medical cannabis improved symptoms of Parkinson's with no adverse effects.[64] A more recent 2023 study from the same journal showed 87 percent of Parkinson's patients saw a reduction in their Parkinson's symptoms, including:[65]

- cramping/dystonia
- pain
- spasticity
- lack of appetite
- dyskinesia
- tremor

In the context of Alzheimer's and Parkinson's, the dialogue extends to the real-world implications of these findings. Certified cannabis nurse Cheri Sacks, RN, CDCES, recounted how, for a patient grappling with Parkinson's, a balanced CBD to THC tincture offered respite from pain and spasms: "The one thing that works to relieve some of the pain is a [cannabis] tincture, one to one, CBD to THC."

In the case of neurodegenerative disorders, cannabis is not a panacea but a valuable adjunct to established therapies. Cannabinoids can provide symptomatic relief across a spectrum of conditions. In Alzheimer's, cannabis can help with agitation, insomnia, anxiety, and appetite stimulation, while offering relief from spasticity and tremors for Parkinson's patients.

Clinical studies and evidence

Clinical studies and research evidence are fundamental pillars in the evaluation of cannabis therapy for neurological disorders. Dr. Kogan emphasizes the necessity of scientific validation in medical decision-making:

> "Right now it's still trial and error for the most part. Funding for these studies is limited, and they get done on a very limited scale based on just doctors like me trying to do something first."

Nonetheless, recent research has provided valuable insights into the efficacy of cannabis-based treatments. For instance, a study in *Frontiers in Physiology* showed a significant reduction in neuropathic pain and improved quality of life in multiple sclerosis patients using cannabinoids.[66] In epilepsy management, a study published in *Scientific Reports* revealed a 50 percent or greater reduction in seizure frequency with CBD treatment in pediatric patients.[67]

As such, clinical trials focusing on cannabis therapy have shown promise in various neurological conditions. Another study published in *Spinal Cord Series and Cases* in 2019 found that cannabis use was associated with reduced pain and improved quality of life in individuals with spinal cord injury.[68] The study also found that cannabis use was associated with improved sleep quality and reduced anxiety and depression.

Patient experiences and case studies

Exploring patient experiences and case studies on the use of cannabis for neurological diseases opens up a complex landscape of individual responses and outcomes. Healthcare professionals who work with medical marijuana often encounter a range of symptoms and challenges unique to neurological conditions.

Dr. Kogan observes:

"In Canada when we took Parkinson's as a challenge, it was clear that patients came to the clinic trying to address the tremor, which was what conditioned them the most. As doctors, we tried to reduce the frequency of the tremor over time, generally using balanced varieties, that is, one part THC, one part CBD."

This approach, while innovative, offers varied success rates, especially when cannabis is administered through inhalation.

Nevertheless, the impact of cannabis on neurological diseases extends beyond treating a single symptom, such as tremors. Dr. Kogan found that the overall quality of life for patients often improved, even if the tremors remained unchanged:

"We saw that the improvement or the impact this had on Parkinson's and the tremor wasn't that significant. But when we surveyed, we conducted a the quality of life survey. We saw that the patient would say phrases like 'I don't know if the tremor improved much, but I feel better, doctor.'"

Moreover, the challenge of addressing the autoimmune aspects of certain neurological conditions, characterized by inflammatory processes, becomes apparent. The modulation and regulation of inflammation through cannabis use present a promising avenue for potentially slowing disease progression by mitigating cytokine release. Dr. Kogan noted the balance between scientific exploration and practical application: "In this daily struggle of basic science and applied science, cannabis works."

Given all of this, it is clear that the benefits of cannabis therapy extend well beyond symptom management, offering potential improvements in overall quality of life for individuals navigating the complexities of neurological conditions.

Risks and challenges

In the exploration of cannabis as a therapeutic option for neurological disorders, we encounter both promise and caution. While it is clear that cannabis holds significant therapeutic potential, it also requires careful consideration and management to handle its challenges effectively.

One of the foremost challenges in incorporating cannabis into treatment regimens for neurological disorders is managing the side effects associated with its use. Research published in the *Journal of Clinical Medicine Research* pinpoints the dual nature of cannabis therapy in chronic pain patients, where alongside pain relief, individuals may experience dizziness, fatigue, and cognitive impairment. The critical need for vigilant monitoring of patients undergoing cannabis therapy to identify and address potential adverse effects promptly is more than evident.[69]

Similarly, a systematic review in *Epilepsy & Behavior* sheds light on the use of CBD in pediatric patients with refractory epilepsy. While CBD has shown promise in reducing seizure frequency, it is not without side effects such as fatigue, diarrhea, and changes in appetite. If progress is to be made in this field, understanding and managing the side effects of cannabis-based treatments to enhance their safety and tolerability for patients with neurological disorders is key.[70]

Amid these challenges, the voices of healthcare professionals resonate with experience and caution. Cheri Sacks articulates a common barrier encountered in the therapeutic use of cannabis— patient fear and misunderstanding, often exacerbated by the recreational market's emphasis on high-THC products. She highlights the importance of education and understanding in overcoming these obstacles:

"That's my number one barrier. And I'm still trying to figure out how to get over the fear. It's real and it happens because they don't understand."

On her part, Dr. Monica Werkheiser recounts a patient's experience to illustrate the importance of cautious, informed decision-making:

"He had been using the product, and it was successful, so he cut and stopped his seizure medication. Cold turkey. Ended up with a seizure because of the withdrawal from the medication."

Another story Dr. Werkheiser shares further illustrates the complexities of cannabinoid therapy in epilepsy:

"I had another patient who was epileptic and had been controlled, seizure free . . . He decided, 'Well, I had more THC, so that must be better.' He decided to cut out the CBD and go straight to THC."

The outcome, unfortunately, was predictable:

"He had been seizure-free for six months, and we had to start at point one again."

This compendium of cases calls attention to the critical need for professional guidance and close monitoring of the use of cannabis for epilepsy. Not to be taken lightly, they vividly illustrate the dangers of uninformed alterations to treatment regimens, emphasizing the essential role of specialists in navigating the therapeutic use of cannabis in neurodegenerative diseases.

Future directions in research and treatment

As the medical field advances, the exploration of cannabis-based therapies for neurological disorders stands at the forefront of

promising research avenues. Dr. Monica Werkheiser sees paral-
lels between the potential of cannabinoids and the multifaceted
approach used in treating HIV/AIDS. Just as a mix of medications
targets different aspects of HIV/AIDS, a similar strategy could be
employed with cannabis to tackle various facets of neurological
disorders:

> "We do this with HIV/AIDS cocktails, where a combination of
> medicines working in different parts of the body is now put
> into products. This is something that is being done in cannabis
> and can be done."

Furthermore, she emphasizes the importance of the convergence of
agriculture and modern medicine, challenging researchers to har-
monize these two fields in developing new therapeutic products.

Additional insight into the practical application of cannabis in
neurological care is provided by Dr. Marcelo Morante, who points
to a promising shift in inpatient treatment strategies. He observes
that patients engaging with cannabis therapies often reduce their
dependence on opioids and benzodiazepines—medications known
for their long-term adverse effects. Dr. Morante suggests that this
trend not only reflects the therapeutic potential of cannabis but also
signals a move towards more holistic treatment methods, stating:

> "Patients who connect with cannabis can save on opioids, save
> on benzodiazepines, offering a glimpse into safer, long-term
> treatment options."

Looking towards the future, Dr. Kogan envisions medical marijuana becoming a cornerstone in the management of neurodegenerative diseases. He acknowledges that while cannabis alone
may not cure conditions such as Alzheimer's disease, its integration into a comprehensive treatment regime could significantly
enhance patient care. The call for further research to fine-tune
cannabinoid profiles, administration methods, and safety meas-
ures is a testament to the dedication of the medical community
to harness cannabis's therapeutic potential fully. Currently, the
path forward offers exciting prospects for the management and
treatment of neurological conditions.

Conclusion

Dr. Kogan, Dr. Werkheiser, Cheri Sacks, RN, and others bring into focus the careful blend of pushing science forward and making a real difference in the lives of those with neurological conditions, through the lens of cannabis treatment. From reducing seizures in epilepsy to easing symptoms in multiple sclerosis and neuro-degenerative diseases, cannabis has shown promise in a variety of contexts.

The narrative that unfolds within these depictions is one of cautious optimism. The remarkable stories of individuals like Charlotte Figi, who found relief from severe epilepsy, accentuate the potential benefits of medical marijuana. Yet, as we've seen, the path forward is not without its hurdles. The challenges of navigating side effects, the need for personalized treatment plans, and the complexities of integrating cannabis with traditional medical approaches remind us that this field is still in its infancy.

The importance of continued research cannot be overstated. As Dr. Kogan suggested, understanding the intricacies of how cannabis interacts with neurological conditions is crucial for its development into a mainstream treatment option. The call for more comprehensive studies and the development of precise treatment protocols reflect a shared commitment to unlocking the full potential of cannabis responsibly and effectively.

The exploration of cannabis in neurological care opens up new avenues for treatment, offering hope and new possibilities for those affected by these conditions. But it also calls for a balanced approach, one that weighs the evidence, acknowledges the challenges, and moves forward with a commitment to patient safety and well-being. As we look to the future, the ongoing dialogue between research, clinical practice, and patient experiences will continue to shape the landscape of cannabis therapy in neurology, driving towards more effective and compassionate care solutions.

7

Mental health and cannabis

This chapter explores the complex relationship between cannabis and mental health in treating conditions like anxiety, depression, and post-traumatic stress disorder (PTSD). It advocates for a balanced approach, emphasizing the importance of caution and personalized treatment in the evolving landscape of cannabis and mental healthcare.

For centuries, cannabis has been used for medicinal purposes, including the management of mental health conditions such as anxiety, depression, and PTSD.[71] In the past few years, interest in the potential use of cannabis as a treatment for mental health disorders has increasingly grown. This chapter will provide an overview of the intersection between mental health and cannabis use, exploring the potential benefits and risks of using medical marijuana to manage mental health conditions.

The potential benefits of using cannabis for mental health treatment are multifaceted and have been the subject of extensive research. Cannabis has been shown to have potential efficacy in reducing anxiety and depression symptoms. Besides, CBD has been suggested to possess antidepressant, anxiolytic, and procognitive properties.[72]

A study published in the *Journal of Affective Disorders* found that cannabis use was associated with a significant reduction in symptoms of depression, anxiety, and stress.[73] Likewise, another study published in the same journal found that cannabis use was associated with a significant reduction in symptoms of PTSD.[74]

However, it is important to consider the risks associated with using marijuana for mental health treatment. Heavy cannabis use has been associated with an increased risk for psychiatric disorders, including psychosis, depression, and anxiety.[75] These risks demand a cautious and evidence-based approach to using cannabis in mental health treatment.

Cannabis and anxiety disorders

Anxiety disorders are a prevalent mental health condition, affecting millions of people worldwide. According to the WHO, they are among the world's most common mental health conditions, affecting 301 million people around the globe in 2019.[76] In the USA alone, an estimated 19.1 percent of adults experience symptoms of anxiety disorder every year.[77]

Anxiety is a stress reaction, and it is a normal and often healthy emotion. However, when a person regularly feels disproportionate levels of anxiety, it might become a medical condition.[78] Anxiety disorders are characterized by excessive and persistent fear and worry about everyday situations. Symptoms of anxiety often manifest during childhood or adolescence, and they may be difficult to control, cause significant distress, and can last a long time if untreated. As such, anxiety disorders interfere with daily activities and can impair a person's family, social, and school or working life.

Nevertheless, cannabis can help manage anxiety by reducing the activity in the amygdala, the part of the brain responsible for the fight or flight response.[79] Dr. Abrams explains that "many of [his] AIDS patients were benefiting from using cannabis, both recreationally and medically, to decrease their anxiety and depression. And also marijuana was very effective in dealing with the nausea generated by the medicines that we gave to treat the virus."

Dr. Paloma Lehfeldt shared her experience involving a patient with generalized anxiety disorder. The patient initially used CBD to manage her symptoms, but when it became less effective, she added another cannabinoid to her regimen, called CBG (cannabigerol). This addition significantly decreased her anxiety disorders.

However, it is essential to approach the use of cannabis for anxiety with caution, as excessive use can lead to increased anxiety and paranoia.[80] The endocannabinoid system plays a crucial role in responses to stress and anxiety, and the two primary active ingredients of cannabis, THC and CBD, have differing effects concerning this condition. Pure THC appears to decrease anxiety at lower doses and increase anxiety at higher doses, while CBD appears to decrease anxiety at all doses that have been tested so far, according to the study "Effects of Marijuana on Mental Health: Anxiety Disorders" by Susan A. Stoner, Ph.D., Research Consultant from the Alcohol & Drug Abuse Institute at the University of Washington, published in June 2017.[81]

Cannabis and depression

According to the WHO, depression is a common mental health condition that affects approximately 280 million people world-wide, including 5 percent of the world's adults.[82] In the USA, an estimated 17.3 million adults, or about 7.1 percent of the US population age 18 and older, experience major depressive disorder in any given year.[83]

Depression is about 50 percent more common among women than among men globally and often co-occurs with other illnesses and medical conditions. For instance, 25 percent of cancer patients experience depression, while 10–27 percent of post-stroke patients struggle with it as well.[84] This condition can lead to problems at school and work, and it can affect all aspects of life, including relationships with family, friends, and community.

A study featured in the *Journal of Affective Disorders* investigated the immediate effects of cannabis use on symptoms of depression, anxiety, and stress, employing data from 11,953 sessions recorded via the Strainprint app, where users document symptom changes post-cannabis consumption.[85] Findings suggest cannabis leads to a 50 percent reduction in depression and a 58 percent reduction in anxiety and stress levels. While smaller doses of inhaled cannabis are enough to alleviate depression and anxiety, the management of stress requires a higher intake. Interestingly, high CBD/low THC cannabis showed the most significant benefit for depression, while high CBD/high THC was best for stress relief. Despite these positive short-term effects, the study noted a potential exacerbation of baseline depression symptoms with ongoing use, without evidence of developing tolerance to cannabis's perceived effects.

Dr. Paloma Lehfeldt, who specializes in cannabis and mental health, explains:

"CBD also affects that serotonin neurotransmitter. It works on the 5-HT1A receptor and raises serotonin in our brains. So it has similar effects to SSRI, but it doesn't take two weeks to take effect. It works much quicker, and it doesn't have the same side effects."

Dr. Lehfeldt notes the similarity in action between cannabinoids and SSRIs (Selective Serotonin Reuptake Inhibitors), explaining that cannabis "affects neurotransmitters in a similar way to SSRIs, which are commonly prescribed for these conditions."

SSRIs are a class of drugs typically used to treat depression and anxiety disorders by increasing the levels of serotonin in the brain, thereby enhancing mood and emotion regulation.

Nevertheless, they are far from being a panacea, as Dr. Lehfeldt explains:

"SSRIs work by increasing serotonin levels, but they're not effective for everyone and come with various side effects, including mood alterations and an increased risk of suicide in younger people. They also take weeks to show effects, which can be detrimental for those suffering from acute anxiety or depression. CBD, like SSRIs, influences serotonin but works more quickly and without the same side effects."

Additionally, CBD has been shown to have antidepressant-like properties in animal models at certain doses. However, more research is needed to determine the optimal dose and duration of CBD treatment for depression.

As previously stated, the use of cannabis for depression should be approached with caution, as excessive use can lead to an increased risk of mental health conditions for some individuals. A review of observational and epidemiological studies found that cannabis use was associated with a modest increased risk for developing depressive symptoms. Yet, the review also found that depression may lead to the onset of or increase in cannabis use frequency.[86]

A meta-analysis of over 76,000 individuals found that cannabis use was associated with a modest increased risk for developing depressive symptoms and that heavy cannabis use was associated with a stronger, but still moderate, increased risk for developing depression.[87] A study published in *Advances in Experimental Medicine and Biology* found that the association between cannabis use and depression may be stronger among men during adolescence and emerging adulthood and stronger in women during midlife.[88] There is also an indication for potential genetic correlation contributing to the comorbidity of cannabis use disorder and depression, namely that serotonin (5-HT) may mediate such association.

Furthermore, the prevalence of major depressive disorder (MDD) in those with cannabis dependence (CD), cannabis use disorder (CUD), and cannabis abuse (CA) is approximately 6.9 percent, 4.7 percent, and 1.0 percent, respectively.[89] This highlights the importance of exploring the relationship between recreational, medical, and heavy cannabis use (including CUD) and depression.

PTSD and cannabis therapy

Post-traumatic stress disorder is a mental health condition that can develop after experiencing or witnessing a traumatic event. Approximately 6 percent of the U.S. population, which translates to around 6 in every 100 people, will experience PTSD at some point in their lives. It's important to note that many individuals with this condition may recover after treatment and no longer fulfill the criteria for PTSD, so this figure includes anyone who may have the disorder during their lifetime, regardless of symptom resolution. Annually, about 5 percent of American adults, or 5 in every 100, are affected by PTSD, amounting to approximately 13 million individuals in 2020 alone. Gender plays a significant role in its prevalence, with women being more susceptible than men. Specifically, about 8 percent of women and 4 percent of men are likely to develop PTSD during their lifetime. This discrepancy is partly attributed to the higher likelihood of women encountering certain types of trauma, such as sexual assault.[90]

This condition can be triggered by a variety of traumatic events, such as military combat, natural disasters, serious accidents, and physical or sexual assault. Symptoms of PTSD can include flashbacks, nightmares, severe anxiety, and uncontrollable thoughts about the event. Said symptoms can be severe and persistent, and can significantly impact a person's ability to function in their daily life.

Research has explored the potential therapeutic use of cannabis and synthetic cannabinoids for improving PTSD symptoms, such as reducing anxiety, modulating memory-related processes, and improving sleep.[91]

However, note that the use of cannabis-based pharmaceuticals containing specified concentrations of specific cannabinoids may have different effects compared to the use of whole-plant cannabis. Research has consistently demonstrated that individuals with PTSD have greater availability of cannabinoid type 1 (CB1) receptors and that cannabis use by individuals with PTSD could produce short-term reductions in PTSD symptoms. Nevertheless, it is also possible that functional problems related to cannabis use, rather than a neurobiological effect of cannabis, might impact PTSD treatment effectiveness.

The science behind cannabis and mental health

Mental health conditions such as anxiety, depression, and PTSD affect millions of people worldwide and can be debilitating and interfere with daily life. And while cannabis has shown potential benefits in managing symptoms of these conditions, the scientific evidence on how this plant affects mental health is still evolving.

One of the most popular cannabinoids found in cannabis is CBD, which has been shown to have relaxing properties. Dr. Patricia Frye, an MD and expert in cannabis science and medicine, explains: "CBD and THC are antioxidant and neuroprotective properties. When combined they are more effective than THC alone addressing various conditions."

As such, CBD works as an effective anti-inflammatory and muscle relaxant, while reducing anxiety and stress. It is also helpful in treating both inflammatory and neuropathic pain, as well as other symptoms that are fueled by inflammation. Additionally, CBD is not impairing, making it a great medicine for patients who need relief without the psychotropic effects of THC.

THC, on the other hand, is the main psychotropic cannabinoid found in cannabis. It has been used for many years to treat a variety of conditions, including sleep disorders, seizures, pain, migraines, and PMS. However, THC also has intoxicating properties, which limit its use as medicine for some patients. Furthermore, about 9 percent of people who use high-THC cannabis can develop a use disorder. Other than that, the adverse effects are very limited and mild, and none of them is considered serious. THC is still a valuable cannabinoid for patients who need relief from chronic disease and chronic discomfort.

However, the hard evidence linking cannabis and improved mental health outcomes is distinctly mixed. A meta-analysis published in the *Lancet Psychiatry* included 83 available studies that, in total, looked at data from over six thousand participants. It found "scarce evidence" that cannabinoids helped their depression, anxiety, ADHD, PTSD, or psychosis.[92]

The risks and challenges of cannabis use in mental health

According to Dr. Paloma Lehfeldt, when considering using cannabis for your mental health, approach it with caution, particularly if you have a history of psychosis or bipolar disorder. THC can exacerbate symptoms in individuals with these conditions. Additionally, if you have a first-degree relative with either of these mental health disorders, also tread carefully while considering cannabis use, as it can unmask these symptoms.

Dr. Frye shared her perspective on the risks of cannabis use, particularly the challenges associated with dosing. She explains that improper dosing can lead to adverse effects, such as giddiness, sleepiness, or what is colloquially referred to as "couch lock." She discusses the potential for dependence or addiction to cannabis, emphasizing that while some individuals may develop a use disorder, the adverse effects are limited, mild, and not considered serious. She also notes that the quality of addiction to cannabis is not the same as the addiction to opiates.

Legal and ethical considerations

Legal and ethical considerations are crucial when it comes to using cannabis for mental health treatment, given that the legal status of the plant and its derivatives varies widely across different countries and states, making it difficult for patients and health-care providers to navigate the system.

Dr. Patricia Frye believes that the medical cannabis programs have been hijacked by the adult use/recreational market:

> "There's so much focus on high THC in those programs that there's very little effort put into formulating things like a nasal spray, which has a great onset of action, just like inhalation."

In this regard, Dr. Mikhail Kogan, a physician and medical canna-bis expert, emphasizes the importance of cultural awareness and patient autonomy when it comes to using cannabis for mental health treatment:

> "The patient's rights and autonomy trump the science . . . it doesn't matter what the science shows. If the particular patient made a choice, most physicians nowadays will accept that."

Conclusion

Wrapping up our journey through the delicate landscape of mental health and cannabis, cannabis presents itself as a complex character in the ongoing story of how we understand and treat mental health disorders. The anecdotal warmth and the cautious optimism of researchers illuminate a path forward that is as intricate as the human mind itself.

The chapters of research and lived experiences weave together a narrative that cannabis, with its symphony of compounds like THC and CBD, presents real opportunities for research into alternative treatments for anxiety, depression, and PTSD. These aren't just conditions, they're profound human experiences that touch millions, and for some, cannabis has been a lantern in the dark.

Yet, as we traverse this promising terrain, we also navigate a minefield of potential risks and legal dilemmas. Cannabis isn't a simple solution. It's a substance that demands respect for its power and its limitations. The stories of those who've found solace in cannabis are tempered by cautionary tales that remind us of the need for a balanced, informed approach.

In this evolving conversation, personal stories and scientific research converge to highlight the importance of a tailored approach to treatment. Cannabis doesn't offer a one-size-fits-all answer but instead poses a question: How can we best harness its potential in a way that is safe, effective, and respectful of individual needs?

The future of cannabis in mental health treatment is unwritten, inviting more research, more dialogue, and more understanding. As we turn the page, let's carry forward the lessons learned and the questions unearthed, embracing both the hope and the challenges that cannabis presents. It's a journey worth taking, with every step forward illuminated by the collective endeavor to improve mental health care for all.

8

Cannabis for sleep disorders

This chapter delves into the potential of cannabis in treating sleep disorders, highlighting the role of cannabinoids like THC, CBD, and CBN in improving sleep quality and duration. It presents research findings and expert opinions on how these compounds interact with sleep mechanisms, offering insights into their benefits and risks.

This chapter aims to provide a comprehensive understanding of cannabis therapy for sleep disorders, emphasizing the need for personalized treatment approaches and further research to optimize therapeutic outcomes.

Cannabis and sleep disorders

Sleep disorders encompass a range of conditions that affect the quality, duration, and timing of sleep, leading to significant disruptions in daily functioning and overall well-being. Scientifically, sleep disorders are defined as conditions that interfere with the normal sleep–wake cycle, encompassing issues like insomnia, sleep apnea, and narcolepsy. According to the American Sleep Apnea Association, it is estimated that approximately 50 to 70 million adults in the USA alone suffer from some form of sleep disorder.[93]

Recently, research studies have shown that cannabinoids, such as THC, CBD, and CBN, can influence sleep patterns by affecting neurotransmitter release, particularly in brain regions involved in sleep regulation. THC, in particular, has been linked to sedative effects that may promote sleep onset but potentially disrupt the later stages of sleep, such as REM (rapid eye movement) sleep. On the other hand, CBD, a non-intoxicating cannabinoid, has shown promise in improving sleep quality and reducing symptoms of insomnia in some individuals.

In the most comprehensive study to date that investigated medical cannabis and insomnia, folks who struggled with sleep were given a combination of THC, CBN, and CBD (20:2:1 ratio).[94] Participants slept on average 33 minutes a night longer, and they were awake 10 minutes less each night compared to the placebo group. Additionally, they reported feeling better rested post-sleep and that they had gotten a better night's sleep.

The interaction between cannabis and sleep disorders is complex and multifaceted, with individual responses varying based on factors such as dosage, timing of administration, and the specific cannabinoid profile of the product used. While some studies suggest a potential benefit of cannabis in managing certain sleep disorders, further research is needed to elucidate the long-term effects and optimal therapeutic strategies.

Cannabis and sleep: Understanding the connection

Insomnia and other sleep disorders are some of the most popular reasons people turn to cannabis as a potential medical treatment method. In fact, some studies show this number to be as high as 47 percent.[95] However, the relationship between cannabis and sleep is certainly complex. Cannabinoids such as THC and CBD have shown promise in offering therapeutic potential for various sleep disorders, a potential underpinned by both scientific research and clinical observations.

CBD promotes sleep by affecting adenosine levels in the central nervous system. According to Dr. Frye, "CBD is a really good medicine for sleep. THC can be helpful, but CBD interacts with that adenosine, which helps to bring on that drowsy, sleepy feeling." This mechanism of action suggests that CBD could serve as a potent sleep aid, enhancing the body's natural sleep processes without the psychoactive effects associated with THC.

However, the conversation around cannabis's potential benefits extends beyond a simple sleep aid. The endocannabinoid system interacts with critical neurotransmitter systems like GABA and serotonin, both vital to sleep regulation. In addition, Dr. Wilson-King calls cannabis a great "potential therapeutic agent for conditions including mood pain, poor sleep, and/or hormonal dysfunction."

This perspective widens the scope of cannabis's clinical application, suggesting its benefits could extend to tackling various conditions that intersect with sleep issues.

Moreover, Dr. Chanda Macias's observations from her experience further cement cannabis's therapeutic potential: "I've seen people make all types of improvements from sleeping at night to being able to go on a jog or swim."

CBN and sleep

CBN is a compound found in the cannabis plant, a cousin of the more famous THC and CBD. But CBN is different. It's what THC becomes when exposed to light and air over time. Think of it as the wise elder of cannabis compounds, offering a gentle nudge towards relaxation and sleep rather than a psychoactive punch.

Recent studies have shed a light on CBN's potential as a sleep aid.[96] Unlike its relatives, CBN doesn't aim to dazzle you with a high or even significantly alter your state of mind. Instead, it's like a whisper telling your body it's time to wind down and rest.

CBN: Alone or with a friend?

While the solo act of CBN is impressive, researchers wondered if pairing it with CBD, another non-psychoactive cannabis compound known for promoting relaxation, would create a super-group for sleep. However, the addition of CBD didn't seem to make a significant difference. It appears CBN doesn't need a backup singer; it can hold the stage on its own when it comes to improving sleep quality.

A nod to safety

One of the sweetest parts of the CBN lullaby is its safety tune. Participants in these studies reported only mild side effects, such as feeling a bit groggy in the morning. But let's be honest, who hasn't felt that way after trying a new sleep aid? The key here is that CBN doesn't seem to cause any serious side effects, making it a potentially safer alternative to other sleep medications that can leave you feeling like you've been hit by a sleeping truck the next day.

Patient experiences

Mara Gordon's involvement in conducting clinical trials on sleep disorders is an example of the importance of rigorous research in understanding the effects of cannabis on sleep. She mentions that "we've even done clinical trials on a human double-blind placebo using a formula that I created."

For many battling sleep disorders, the journey to slumber is fraught with obstacles, and cannabis may offer a glimmer of hope. Mara Gordon emphasizes the prevalence of sleep issues and the necessity of a customized cannabis treatment plan, suggesting that "if somebody's got a sleep disorder, which is so incredibly common, I would usually get them around 15 milligrams of THC."

Dr. Morante's account further illuminates cannabis's transformative impact, especially for those suffering from PTSD and chronic pain:

> "Many patients who used cannabis found this improvement in sleep structure which, when one treats post-traumatic stress disorder, greatly improved mood and appetite. One could go on reducing medications that one usually uses, such as benzodiazepines, antidepressants."

On a similar note, Dr. Grinspoon reflects that shifting patients from opiates to cannabis often leads to a better "quality of life" and sleep improvement. This testament to cannabis's potential highlights the significant shift away from traditional medications.

Risks and side effects

THC's psychoactive properties can offer both solace and challenge. While many find THC effective in inducing sleep and reducing nighttime wakenings, there's a flip side to its use. As highlighted by Dr. Duclas Charles, THC's potential to "actually make anxiety worse or exacerbate it" (see Chapter 8) cannot be overlooked. This risk is particularly pertinent for individuals with sleep disorders intertwined with anxiety, such as PTSD patients, where the goal is to soothe the mind rather than stimulate it.

CBD's emergence as a therapeutic ally in cannabis medicine offers a less fraught path for patients, particularly those dealing with sleep disorders. Its non-psychotropic nature and potential for reducing anxiety and promoting relaxation make CBD an attractive option. Dr. Frye's remarks on the mild nature of CBD's adverse effects highlight its suitability, especially for patients cautious of THC's risks. This safety profile, coupled with CBD's therapeutic versatility, positions it as a cornerstone in the treatment of sleep disorders, offering relief without the heightened risk of adverse psychological effects.

Mara Gordon's advice on starting with low doses of cannabis, especially when targeting sleep disorders, emphasizes the need for a prudent approach to minimizing risks. This strategy is crucial not only in avoiding the potential exacerbation of anxiety with THC but also in fine-tuning the dose for individual efficacy and comfort (for more on dosage see Chapter 11). Her reassurance that the effects of overconsumption are temporary and manageable without long-term repercussions offers comfort to patients experimenting with dosages to find their therapeutic sweet spot.

Conclusion

In wrapping up our dive into how cannabis can be a game-changer for those tossing and turning at night, it's clear that this isn't just about getting high. It's about understanding a plant that's been around the block—a plant that, according to Dr. Patricia Frye, demands respect for its nuanced benefits. She puts it simply and powerfully:

> "It's an amazing plant and it deserves a lot of respect. The cannabinoids target all of the things that come along with chronic pain. CBD is a great anxiolytic, meaning it reduces anxiety. It can be mood-elevating. THC at low doses is also a good anxiolytic and it lowers anxiety. Both CBD and THC are muscle-relaxing. THC is mood-elevating. And CBD can be very helpful for sleep. THC can too. But you know when we use Dronabinol, which is the THC molecule just suspended in sesame oil, I don't

get a lot of feedback from patients that they have sleepiness during the day the way DBS does. DBS works by a mechanism in the brain that helps people to become drowsy and drift into sleep more readily."

This isn't just a superficial endorsement, it's a call to look deeper into how these natural compounds can genuinely make life better for those struggling to find rest at night.

We've wandered through the science, listened to what the docs say, and heard straight from those who've been in the trenches with insomnia, sleep apnea, and all those gremlins that steal sleep. The big takeaway? THC, CBD, and CBN each play their parts in the sleep saga. THC might help you nod off, but it's a bit of a double-edged sword depending on how much you take. CBD, on the other hand, is like the cool uncle—helpful, without getting you buzzed. And then there's CBN, the quiet achiever, promising a smoother slide into dreamland.

This journey through cannabinoids has shown us that the role cannabis can play in fighting sleep disorders is layered, potent, and full of promise. From reducing nighttime wake-ups to easing the mind, the potential benefits are as varied as they are significant. It's not just about finding a quick fix but understanding how different strains and doses can tailor-fit a solution to what keeps each of us up at night.

Of course, it's not all roses and sunshine. THC has its quirks, potentially ramping up anxiety for some, making it clear that one size does not fit all. This is where CBD steps up as the milder, gentler option for those wary of getting too high or too anxious. It's about striking a balance, starting low and going slow, and always keeping the dialogue open with healthcare providers who are finally beginning to see cannabis not as a last resort but as a viable first step.

So, as we close the chapter on cannabis and sleep, the message is clear: there's hope on the horizon for the sleep-deprived. It's not just about catching more Zs but enhancing the quality of life for those who've just about tried everything else. As research continues to evolve, so too will our understanding and appreciation for how cannabis, in all its complexity, can be a cornerstone in not just managing sleep disorders but potentially transforming lives for the better.

9

Cannabis and glaucoma

This chapter explores the potential of cannabis in treating glaucoma, focusing on its ability to lower intraocular pressure, a key factor in the disease's progression. It delves into the challenges of implementing cannabis-based treatments, including dosing, side effects, and regulatory hurdles.

Highlighting expert insights and patient experiences, the chapter advocates for continued research to optimize cannabis therapies for glaucoma, emphasizing the importance of a nuanced approach to treatment and the need for advancements in legal and ethical frameworks.

What is glaucoma?

Glaucoma, a group of eye conditions characterized by damage to the optic nerve and gradual vision loss, is a leading cause of irreversible blindness worldwide. Medically, glaucoma is defined as a progressive optic neuropathy that results in peripheral vision loss. Globally, it is estimated that over 60 million people are affected by glaucoma, making it a significant public health concern.

The role of cannabis in the treatment of glaucoma stems from its ability to lower intraocular pressure (IOP), a key risk factor for the development and progression of the disease. Studies have demonstrated that cannabinoids, particularly THC, can effectively reduce IOP by enhancing the outflow of aqueous humor from the eye or decreasing its production. This pressure-lowering effect is attributed to the activation of cannabinoid receptors in the eye, which regulate the balance of fluid dynamics and help maintain a healthy optic nerve function.

Despite the promising results of early research on cannabis and glaucoma, challenges remain in translating these findings into clinically approved treatments. Issues such as dosing precision, potential side effects, and regulatory constraints pose hurdles to the widespread adoption of cannabis-based therapies for glaucoma.

Continued investigation into the mechanisms of action, safety profile, and long-term efficacy of cannabis in glaucoma management is essential for advancing our understanding and improving patient outcomes.

Treating glaucoma with cannabis

Glaucoma has long been a focus of research exploring alternative treatments beyond traditional medications and surgeries.

As previously stated, the potential of medical marijuana in managing glaucoma has sparked interest due to its ability to influence IOP. However, understanding the nuances of using cannabis for glaucoma treatment requires a comprehensive examination of the scientific evidence, potential benefits, and inherent limitations.

THC lowers IOP, but the relief is often temporary and lasts 2 to 3 hours. However, CBD can raise IOP, so people with glaucoma need to be careful and see their eye doctor to have their pressures checked if they're considering medical marijuana as an avenue of treatment.

Dr. Monica Werkheiser shares a critical perspective on cannabis as a treatment. "It's a fallacy to think that cannabis is going to treat your glaucoma . . . It's not a sustained relief, which is the issue."

As such, despite the promising effects of THC on intraocular pressure, the sustainability and long-term efficacy of cannabis in treating glaucoma remain subjects of debate and concern.

Clinical research and trials

In the realm of clinical research and trials exploring the therapeutic potential of cannabinoids for glaucoma, a wealth of scientific evidence and expert insights converge to shed light on the intricate mechanisms and challenges in utilizing cannabis-based interventions for these conditions.

The research landscape on cannabinoids for glaucoma is multifaceted, with studies exploring molecular targets, therapeutic approaches on intraocular pressure, neuroprotective actions, and vascular targets. While evidence suggests a potential role for cannabinoids in lowering intraocular pressure, challenges such as short duration of action, tachyphylaxis (the rapidly diminishing response to successive doses of a drug, rendering it less effective), and systemic side effects pose limitations to their widespread use in glaucoma treatment.

Risks and side effects

The use of cannabis in treating glaucoma presents a promising avenue for patients seeking alternative therapies. However, there are potential risks and side effects associated with cannabis, particularly concerning its psychoactive compounds and the variability in individual response.

THC has been noted for its potential to reduce intraocular pressure, but the intoxicating effects of THC can be disconcerting for some patients, leading to discomfort and, in some cases, exacerbation of anxiety. Thus, weigh the therapeutic benefits of this cannabinoid against the potential for psychological distress. Use a cautious approach in managing glaucoma with cannabis, where the goal is to achieve symptomatic relief without compromising mental well-being. Engage in open dialogue with your healthcare provider about dosing strategies, balancing the potential for intraocular pressure reduction with the need to avoid undue psychoactive effects.

As the medical community delves deeper into the benefits and risks of using cannabis for glaucoma, the emphasis on informed, personalized treatment plans becomes increasingly clear. Understanding the specific challenges and therapeutic goals of each patient allows for a tailored approach that maximizes benefits while minimizing risks.

Educating patients on the nuances of THC and CBD, the importance of cautious dosing, and the variability in individual response is essential. This education empowers patients to make informed decisions about their treatment, fostering a partnership with healthcare providers that hinges on confidence and care.

Legal and ethical issues

Navigating the legal and ethical landscape surrounding the prescription of cannabis for glaucoma involves an intermesh of regulatory frameworks, patient rights, healthcare provider responsibilities, and societal perceptions.

The legal status of cannabis varies across jurisdictions, with some regions permitting medical use under specific conditions, while others maintain strict regulations or prohibitions. Understanding the legal frameworks governing the prescription, distribution, and use of cannabis for medical purposes is essential for healthcare providers, patients, and policymakers alike.

Furthermore, ethical considerations in prescribing cannabis for glaucoma encompass issues of patient autonomy, beneficence, non-maleficence, and justice. Healthcare providers must engage in informed discussions with patients regarding the risks, benefits, alternatives, and uncertainties associated with cannabis therapy, ensuring that decisions align with patient values and preferences.

Providers must respect patient rights, confidentiality, and privacy in the context of cannabis therapy and uphold ethical standards and legal obligations in their practice. Informed consent, shared decision-making, and ongoing monitoring are essential components of patient-centered care when considering cannabis as a treatment option for glaucoma.

Future research and potential therapies

The scene of medical research is continually evolving, with a growing emphasis on exploring the therapeutic potential of cannabis for addressing complex health conditions such as glaucoma.

Dr. Frye's vision for the future of cannabis in healthcare resonates with the need for continued research and innovation:

> "I think that there's going to be more of a trend towards single-molecule medicines. I hope that the pharmaceutical grade products don't strip things down to single-molecule but can manufacture products in ways that will maintain the integrity of the plant."

Emerging therapies involving cannabis focus on targeting specific molecular pathways, neuroprotective mechanisms, and novel drug delivery systems to enhance the efficacy and safety of treatment. Studies have explored the potential of cannabinoids in modulating intraocular pressure, protecting retinal cells, and mitigating neuroinflammation associated with glaucoma progression.

Conclusion

In the realm of glaucoma treatment, cannabis is emerging not just as a compound of interest but as a contender in the ongoing quest for better health solutions. The insights from doctors and researchers shed light on cannabis's nuanced role in medicine, suggesting cautious optimism. This isn't merely about endorsing a new treatment option, but about understanding and navigating its complexities. Cannabis presents a range of possibilities, yet it's accompanied by a suite of considerations—dosage, individual response, and the delicate balance of benefits against potential side effects.

The call for more research is loud and clear, pinpointing the need for a deeper dive into how cannabis can be safely and effectively integrated into treatment regimens. This isn't just a matter of accumulating more data but of pursuing a nuanced understanding of how cannabinoids interact with the human body, and how these interactions can be harnessed for therapeutic benefit.

Legal and ethical discussions add another layer to this exploration, and they touch on broader societal issues. These conversations go beyond the clinical, ranging from patient rights, and access to treatment, to the evolving legal landscape that frames the availability of cannabis-based therapies. Apart from navigating regulatory hurdles, ensuring that advances in medical cannabis are accessible, equitable, and aligned with patient needs and safety is key.

10
Cannabis and inflammatory bowel disease

This chapter discusses the potential of cannabis in treating Inflammatory Bowel Disease (IBD), focusing on its interaction with the endocannabinoid system and the gastrointestinal tract. It covers how cannabinoids may reduce inflammation and manage IBD symptoms, emphasizing personalized treatment approaches.

IBD and cannabis

IBD is a condition that affects millions globally, disrupting lives and challenging the quest for quality of life. The cornerstone of understanding cannabis's potential in this context is the ECS, especially its significant role in gut health and inflammation management as the gut is filled with CB2 receptors that interact with ECS.

IBD blankets life-altering conditions like Crohn's disease and ulcerative colitis, chronic inflammatory disorders that relentlessly attack the gastrointestinal tract, leading to a spectrum of symptoms. For instance, Crohn's disease can manifest anywhere along the digestive tract, while ulcerative colitis primarily affects the colon and rectum. IBD symptoms can range from mild to severe. These symptoms not only fluctuate with unpredictable flare-ups and periods of remission but also profoundly impact daily functioning and quality of life.

Emerging research suggests that cannabinoids hold anti-inflammatory properties that could offer relief to those battling IBD. By modulating the immune system's response in the gut, these components may help reduce inflammation and alleviate some of the debilitating symptoms of IBD. Thus, incorporating cannabis into IBD management opens a promising lane for alternative therapies, offering hope for improved well-being and symptom relief alongside conventional treatments.

Understanding IBD: Crohn's disease and ulcerative colitis

Crohn's disease is a form of IBD that causes inflammation deep within the layers of the intestinal wall. It can affect any part of the gastrointestinal (GI) tract, leading to symptoms such as:

- persistent diarrhea
- abdominal pain
- rectal bleeding
- weight loss
- fatigue

The inflammation in Crohn's disease can occur in patches that are adjacent to healthy tissue, and it may involve complications like abscesses, strictures, and fistulas.[97] Individuals with Crohn's disease may require surgery to remove damaged portions of the gastrointestinal tract when medications no longer provide relief.[98]

On another hand, ulcerative colitis is another type of IBD that primarily affects the colon and rectum. Unlike Crohn's disease, which can involve any part of the GI tract, ulcerative colitis causes continuous inflammation starting at the rectum and extending further into the colon. Common symptoms of ulcerative colitis include:

- abdominal pain
- diarrhea with blood
- urgency to have a bowel movement
- weight loss
- fever
- anemia
- malnutrition[99]

Long-term inflammation in ulcerative colitis can lead to complications like abscesses, strictures, and an increased risk of colon cancer.

Diagnosing IBD involves a combination of:

- endoscopic procedures like colonoscopy or endoscopy
- imaging studies such as MRI or CT scans
- stool samples
- blood tests

Treatment typically includes medications like:

- 5-aminosalicylic acids
- immunomodulators
- corticosteroids
- biologics to control inflammation and manage symptoms
- surgery in severe cases or when medications are ineffective to remove damaged parts of the intestines

Currently, research on IBD continues to explore various aspects of these conditions, such as genetic predisposition, environmental factors that may contribute to its development, the role of the immune system in causing inflammation, and potential treatments to improve outcomes for individuals with Crohn's disease and ulcerative colitis. By delving into these areas through clinical trials and observational studies conducted by healthcare professionals and researchers worldwide, advancements in managing IBD are being made to enhance patient care and quality of life.

Cannabis compounds and IBD

The exploration of cannabinoids in the battle against IBD has encouraged research, sparking hope for countless sufferers. Plenty of IBD patients already treat their symptoms with cannabis, around 10–12 percent according to several studies.[100] Most sought out cannabis for help with pain, nausea, appetite loss, and sleep disturbances. Cannabinoids modulate the gut's motility and can help with pain. For those with IBS or IBD, like Crohn's and colitis, where inflammation causes significant discomfort, cannabinoids offer relief. Studies have shown that people with IBS have malfunctioning CB1 receptors, and introducing CB1 antagonists can slow gastrointestinal movement. Dronabinol, another cannabinoid, has shown to reduce gastric emptying.[101]

The ECS plays a crucial role in regulating the movement and function of immune cells. This regulation helps control inflammation and immune responses, which is especially important for managing conditions like IBD and IBS. The system's influence extends to key bodily systems, including the brain and gastrointestinal tract, highlighting its therapeutic potential in treating these conditions. Additionally, the ECS has vast therapeutic potential due to its presence in key bodily systems, including the brain and gastrointestinal tract.

Meanwhile, Dr. Paloma Lehfeldt points out the promising effects of cannabigerol, a minor cannabinoid, on gut health. CBG is a non-psychotropic cannabis compound known as the "mother of all cannabinoids," due to its role as a precursor from which other cannabinoids are synthesized, and it is gaining attention for its potential to ease inflammation and pain without intoxicating effects.

Clinical studies on cannabis and IBD

The past few years have seen a growing interest in the medical community about the potential of cannabis in treating IBD. This curiosity has sparked numerous clinical studies aiming to unravel the effects of cannabis compounds on IBD symptoms and inflammation.

According to a systematic review published in *Clinical Gastroenterology* that analyzed the results of 20 different studies, cannabis did not cause remission in any of the 146 participants. However, all reported that their clinical symptoms improved with cannabis and patients' hospital stays were shorter for the cannabis and cannabinoid cohorts.[102] These symptoms included:

- abdominal pain
- general well-being
- nausea
- diarrhea
- poor appetite

Dr. Rajiv Sharma encapsulates the optimism surrounding cannabis research, emphasizing the ECS's significant role in modulating inflammation and its broader health implications. He notes that studies about the ECS "have shown that [cannabinoids] decrease inflammation in the body. They also decrease the risk of cancer, decreasing tumor growth, and inducing the destruction of bad cells." Thus, cannabis has shown the potential to provide a multipronged approach to health, encompassing cancer prevention and tumor management.

Expanding on the therapeutic reach of cannabis in gut health, Dr. Morante explains:

"The digestive tract is full of receptors for cannabis, and many of today's chronic anxiety diseases are linked to digestive disorders like colon inflammation, bloating, abdominal pain, and gas. Cannabis, through its digestive route, modulates these receptors and modulates the release of neurotransmitters and even the inflammation that generates that sick digestive tract that, in a way, has a direct communication with the brain."

In addition, Dr. Frye points out the significant findings from studies under Dr. Timna Naftali, gastroenterologist, and leading cannabis researcher:[103]

"Most of the studies on inflammatory bowel disease have come out of Israel in Tel Aviv. Most of those studies show that the patients in the studies who are smoking THC-dominant flower almost always experience symptom relief. So their abdominal pain gets better, and their diarrhea gets better. They're not having bloody stools. They feel better. They have more energy."

However, Dr. Frye also mentions a crucial gap in the research—the lack of observable changes in inflammation via colonoscopies in the short term, indicating an area for future exploration.

Patient perspectives on cannabis for IBD

When discussing IBD treatment, one aspect stands out and deserves further examination: the patients' experiences and their outcomes, particularly when integrating cannabis into their management plans.

By delving into the experiences of patients firsthand, we come to see just how much cannabinoids can change the way we deal with IBD. It's not just about numbers anymore; it's about the actual difference they can make in people's lives.

For instance, Dr. Frye shares compelling anecdotes from her practice. One case involves a 16-year-old who, after struggling with the limitations of conventional medications like Remicade and Humira, found remarkable relief through a CBD and THC regimen, before such treatments were widely accessible:

"He went on to do well; he had decreased abdominal pain, and decreased output, which means decreased diarrhea, blood, and mucus. His nausea got better. He wasn't as stressed out. His appetite improved; his sleeping, and his weight went up. And lo and behold, about two years out from using these cannabinoids, his MRI normalized."

Another patient's experience further supports the therapeutic potential of cannabinoids, with a focus on CBD and CBDA (cannabidiolic acid, a minor cannabinoid), noted for their potent anti-inflammatory properties:

"I have another patient. Same situation, except he didn't use CBD and THC in a 1 to 1 [ratio]. I had him on CBD and CBDA for about 18 months: [after] two years on cannabinoids, his colonoscopy normalized."

Dr. Frye observes that such outcomes might not be widely reported in studies, perhaps due to the methodologies employed, such as smoking, which can introduce its own set of complications. Instead, capsules or oils are a more appropriate method of treatment, particularly for their efficacy in delivering cannabinoids directly to the gut, where they are most needed. Moreover, capsules and oils are more likely to stay in the gut as well.

The stories of these young patients, one of whom overcame a stricture and improved significantly to the point of reversing his ostomy, paint a picture of hope and resilience. Dr. Frye concludes: "He's graduated from high school and is working, living his best life."

Navigating legal and ethical issues

While the therapeutic potential of cannabis for managing IBD is compelling, it's not without associated risks and challenges. The enthusiasm for cannabis as a treatment option must be balanced with consideration and awareness of its side effects, variability in patient responses, and the legal and regulatory environment.

Cannabis, like any therapeutic agent, comes with a spectrum of potential side effects. While many patients tolerate cannabis well, some may experience adverse effects such as dizziness, dry mouth, fatigue, and in some cases, psychological effects, such as anxiety or paranoia, especially with high THC formulations. There are also concerns about the long-term impact of cannabis use on mental health, particularly in young patients or those with a predisposition to mental health disorders.

Moreover, the risk of dependency cannot be overlooked. The National Institute on Drug Abuse notes that marijuana use can lead to cannabis use disorder, which in severe cases can take the form of addiction.[104] This risk underscores the importance of medical supervision and careful patient selection.

One of the significant challenges in using cannabis for IBD treatment is the variability in products and the lack of standardization. The cannabis plant contains hundreds of cannabinoids, terpenes, and flavonoids, which can vary widely from one strain to another and even from one batch to another. This variability can affect the therapeutic efficacy and side effect profile of cannabis products, making it difficult to predict patient responses and ensure consistent treatment outcomes.

On another note, the legal landscape for cannabis use is complex and varies significantly by jurisdiction. In some regions, medical cannabis is legal and regulated, while in others, it remains illegal or heavily restricted. This legal patchwork poses challenges for patients seeking access to cannabis for medical purposes and for healthcare providers looking to prescribe or recommend it as part of a treatment regimen.

Despite the growing body of research into the use of cannabis to treat IBD, significant gaps remain in our understanding of its efficacy, mechanisms of action, and optimal dosing strategies. The current evidence base consists largely of patient-reported outcomes, small-scale studies, and preclinical research, with a need for larger, randomized controlled trials to provide more definitive guidance. The lack of comprehensive clinical guidelines for the use of cannabis in IBD treatment further complicates its integration into patient care. Physicians and patients often navigate this therapeutic option with limited formal guidance, relying on anecdotal evidence or the findings from limited studies.

Given these risks and challenges, patient education and informed consent become paramount. Patients considering cannabis for IBD management should be fully informed about the potential benefits and risks, the variability in cannabis products, and the legal implications of cannabis use. A collaborative approach to decision-making, involving both the patient and the healthcare provider, is essential to this kind of treatment.

Future directions in cannabis research for IBD

As we explore the burgeoning field of cannabis research in the treatment of Inflammatory Bowel Disease, the perspectives and predictions of medical experts like Dr. Rajiv Sharma underscore the complexity of pain perception and its management, a crucial aspect for IBD sufferers. He explains the potential interplay between the ECS, the gut-brain axis, and their combined effect on both the physical and emotional dimensions of pain:

> "The perception of pain lies somewhere at the interface of mind, body, soul . . . And I feel our system has a role in the perception of pain. And I think mostly it affects the physical side of things. But I would not be surprised that, because the brain and the gut have such a strong attraction, cannabis not only minimizes pain at the site of origin of the pain but also the perception of how the brain and the central nervous system process the pain as well."

This holistic view opens several avenues for future inquiry and innovation in the use of cannabis for IBD, setting the stage for a deeper understanding and potentially revolutionary treatment paradigms.

Thus, the potential for personalized cannabis therapies emerges as a critical area for future exploration. Given the variability in how individuals respond to cannabis, tailoring treatments to fit the specific needs and circumstances of each patient could enhance efficacy and minimize side effects. This personalization will likely rely on advancing our understanding of cannabinoid pharmacology, improving the quality and consistency of cannabis-based products, and developing precise dosing guidelines.

Furthermore, Dr. Sharma's reflections prompt a reassessment of research methodologies. There's a growing need for studies that not only track the clinical outcomes of cannabis use in IBD patients but also examine its effects on quality of life and mental health over the long term. Such comprehensive research could provide the evidence needed to integrate cannabis more fully into IBD treatment protocols.

Conclusion

Throughout this chapter, we've traversed the landscape of IBD, a condition marked by its complexity, variability, and profound impact on the lives of millions. The narratives and studies shared here underscore the significant potential of cannabis to offer relief and improve the quality of life for those living with IBD. The critical insights from medical professionals like Dr. Patricia Frye, Dr. Rajiv Sharma, and others not only highlight the therapeutic benefits of cannabinoids like THC, CBD, and CBG but also advocate for a personalized approach to treatment, mindful of the unique needs and responses of each patient.

Patient stories, particularly those shared by Dr. Frye, serve as powerful testimonials to the transformative impact of cannabis on IBD management, revealing the importance of considering both the physiological and psychological dimensions of treatment and the need for a holistic approach that addresses the totality of patient experience.

Yet, as we've discussed, using cannabis in treating IBD brings about its challenges. From the legal and ethical complexities surrounding medical marijuana use to the ongoing debates about its efficacy and safety, the path forward is fraught with questions and considerations. Despite the obstacles, the drive towards understanding and utilizing cannabis in IBD treatment speaks to a broader commitment to innovation, patient care, and the relentless pursuit of better outcomes.

Looking to the future, the potential directions for cannabis research in IBD treatment are vast and varied. For instance, the speculation by Dr. Rajiv Sharma about the interconnectedness of pain perception, the endocannabinoid system, and the gut-brain axis opens new avenues for investigation.

In this dynamic and changing field, the collective efforts of researchers, clinicians, patients, and advocates are essential. Together, they forge the path towards a future where the integration of cannabis into IBD treatment is informed by robust evidence, guided by patient needs, and characterized by a compassionate and comprehensive approach to care.

11

Practical guidance
Using medical cannabis safely

This chapter delves into the safe and effective use of medical cannabis, guided by experts like Dr. Peter Grinspoon, Dr. Patricia Frye and Cheri Sacks, RN, CDCES. It emphasizes the importance of starting with low doses, understanding the roles of THC and CBD, and customizing treatments to individual needs.

The chapter aims to equip readers with knowledge for responsible medical cannabis use, highlighting patient-centric approaches and the importance of precise dosing to minimize side effects and ensure safety, especially for older adults and those exploring cannabis as an alternative to conventional medications.

Understanding the safe and responsible use of medical cannabis is fundamental to its therapeutic application. Key points include the importance of starting with low doses, precise dosing to minimize side effects, and selecting the right cannabis strains and methods for individual health needs. This guidance aims to help readers navigate medical cannabis use responsibly, whether they are new to it or experienced.

The goal according to health professionals is to ensure medical cannabis serves as a valuable part of personalized healthcare, emphasizing safety and patient-centric approaches.

Comprehensive clinical evaluation and prescriptive guidelines

In an integrative and holistic medical approach, healthcare professionals aim to look at you as a whole instead of merely addressing a single symptom. Particularly, cannabis-centered professionals examine how diet, physical activity, stress, and gastrointestinal health affect the endocannabinoid system.

Consultations for individuals interested in cannabinoid therapies involve a thorough clinical evaluation, which can take up
to an hour or more. This approach stands in contrast to the
more rushed appointments in traditional healthcare settings.
Needless to say, prescriptions for cannabinoid products, along
with recommendations for dosage, concentration, and route of
administration, should always come from a qualified healthcare provider, especially for patients with delicate conditions or
chronic illnesses.

Dosing guidelines and strategies: Low and slow

The golden rule for all cannabis users, especially newcomers, is to
"start low and go slow." This approach minimizes adverse effects
and helps you and your provider find the optimal therapeutic
dose for you.

THC can have a relaxing effect, and patients often report that
it helps them cope with anxiety. However, in higher amounts,
THC can sometimes worsen anxiety or exacerbate it. This is
particularly evident when individuals overconsume cannabis.
Therefore, best practices say to find the minimum effective dose
to minimize the risk of adverse side effects.

Dr. Marcelo Morante, a specialist in cannabis for health and
neuroscience, explains:

> "In selecting cannabis as a therapeutic tool, the initial con-
> sideration revolves around the chosen delivery method. For
> instance, if inhalation is opted for, the desired anxiolytic effects
> may manifest within minutes. Conversely, if a digestive route is
> preferred, the onset could extend beyond an hour with a poten-
> tially milder impact and prolonged latency. Therefore, the pri-
> mary focus is on identifying the condition being addressed and
> determining the most suitable delivery mode. Subsequently,
> the formulation becomes paramount. Much like prescribing
> antibiotics, specifying the desired active compounds and their
> respective doses is crucial as it directly influences the therapeu-
> tic outcome. For instance, in treating anxiety disorders often
> associated with insomnia, a balanced 1:1 variety administered
> via inhalation may be recommended."

This approach facilitates rapid onset akin to intravenous administration, fostering regulation within the central nervous system. By alleviating negative effects, patients experience anxiety relief and enhanced sleep quality. Dr. Morante continues:

"Cannabis plays a pivotal role, affecting neurotransmitter release and inflammatory processes from the intestines to the brain. By selecting the appropriate route, we can efficiently influence these key areas, whether swiftly or gradually."

Cheri Sacks, a registered nurse specializing in cannabis digital therapy, uses an approach rooted in the belief that every individual's experience with cannabis is unique, advocating for careful monitoring and adjustment of dosages as needed:

"It's the basics. It doesn't matter what you're using only use a little bit. You can always add more. And you may not feel anything but that's good. It's better not to feel anything than to feel too high."

A brief guide to starting dosing

Table 11.1 Low doses by treatment method

Treatment method	Recommended low dose	Notes
Smoking/vaporizing	1–2 puffs (1–2 mg THC/CBD per puff)	Effects are felt within minutes; start with one puff and wait 15–20 minutes before considering more.
Edibles	2.5–5 mg THC/CBD	Start with a low dose and wait at least 2 hours before consuming more due to delayed onset.
Tinctures	2.5–5 mg THC/CBD (approximately 0.25–0.5 ml depending on concentration)	Effects can be felt within 15-45 minutes. Hold the tincture under the tongue for faster absorption.

(*Continued*)

Table 11.1 (*Continued*)

Treatment method	Recommended low dose	Notes
Capsules	2.5–5 mg THC/CBD	Similar to edibles, effects may take 1–2 hours to onset; start low and monitor the effects.
Topicals	Use a small amount on the affected area	Localized effects; unlikely to produce systemic effects, but start with a small amount to assess tolerance and effectiveness.

Practical guidance for safe use

- **Smoking/vaporizing**: The effects of inhaled cannabis are usually felt within minutes and can last for 2–3 hours. Starting with one puff allows you to gauge your tolerance and avoid overconsumption.
- **Edibles**: These have a delayed onset (up to 2 hours) and can last longer (up to 6–8 hours). It's crucial to wait before taking more to avoid an intense experience.
- **Tinctures**: Administered sublingually (under the tongue), tinctures can provide a more controlled dosage with a relatively quick onset compared to edibles.
- **Capsules**: Like edibles, they have a delayed onset and are ideal for consistent dosing.
- **Topicals**: These are applied directly to the skin and are used for localized relief. They are not psychoactive and are safe for regular use without systemic effects.

Important considerations

- **Individual tolerance**: Each person's reaction to cannabis can vary significantly based on their body chemistry, tolerance levels, and previous experience with cannabis.

- **Product potency**: Always check the product's concentration of THC and CBD. Start with products that have lower concentrations to better manage dosing.
- **Consult with healthcare professionals**: Especially for medical use, it's advisable to consult with a healthcare provider to tailor the dosage to your specific needs and conditions.

THC and CBD ratios and strain selection

Following Dr. Frye's groundwork, Dr. Mikhail Kogan, a leading figure in Integrative Geriatrics and Medical Director of the GW Center for Integrative Medicine, reinforced the safety of medical cannabis, particularly by emphasizing its zero fatality and direct toxicity record. It is suitable for older adults and those seeking pharmaceutical alternatives.

Selecting the right cannabis strain is crucial for safe, effective medical treatment, with an industry now offering seeds specifically bred for a balanced 1:1 CBD to THC ratio. Strains with specific terpenes can further enhance their therapeutic effects.

A 1:1 ratio means that the product contains equal parts of CBD and THC. This balance can offer therapeutic benefits, such as pain relief, without producing overly strong psychoactive effects that can be associated with high THC concentrations. CBD is known for its anti-inflammatory and non-intoxicating properties, while THC can help with pain and spasticity.

This safety factor becomes crucial in the context of older adults, who are disproportionately affected by the side effects of conventional medications. And while the euphoric effects of cannabis might provide respite from chronic disease and discomfort for some, for others, it could result in dysphoria. This variability in response, often due to imprecise dosing, could lead to adverse effects like excessive sedation or "couch lock". This historical perspective sheds light on the necessity of accurate dosing in modern cannabinoid medicine, to harness its benefits while minimizing potential adverse effects.

It's a common misconception that any amount of cannabis consumption leads to euphoria. However, CBD can mitigate some of the intoxicating effects of THC, balancing symptom relief without overwhelming psychoactivity. Sacks explains:

> "By employing precise dosing, particularly through microdosing, one can circumvent this phenomenon. Exceeding tolerance thresholds can lead to euphoria, followed by heightened anxiety exacerbated by THC. Prolonged consumption may escalate to racing thoughts, paranoia, and increased anxiety levels. Educating patients, particularly those with mental health conditions such as PTSD, bipolar disorder, schizophrenia, or severe anxiety, about THC's propensity to induce these symptoms is paramount."

This nuanced approach to cannabinoid ratios is part of her broader strategy to ensure patients receive the most benefit from their cannabis treatment while maintaining a high quality of life.

Today, many cannabis users still believe that THC is what calms them down or helps with anxiety. However, CBD, not THC, plays that role.

CBD and THC compete for the same receptors in the body. If you over-consume THC or experience its side effects like euphoria, higher doses of CBD can potentially counteract those effects or serve as a rescue or antidote.

Dr. Patricia Frye highlights how the medical community's understanding of cannabis, starting with THC and CBD, has evolved significantly. Initially, the euphoric effects of THC were viewed negatively, but these perceptions have shifted as its therapeutic benefits in providing relief from chronic discomfort have become more apparent. Meanwhile, CBD has emerged as a "promiscuous molecule," interacting with numerous receptors, making it beneficial for a wide range of conditions, especially due to its potent anti-inflammatory properties and non-impairing nature. While each has distinct benefits, their combination often leads to more effective treatment outcomes. This synergy evidences the necessity of understanding the nuances of medical cannabis use, including the potential for developing a use disorder with high THC use, albeit relatively low compared to other substances.

CBD, THC, and more

Beyond THC and CBD, the cannabis plant harbors a wealth of lesser-known components such as minor cannabinoids, terpenes, and flavonoids, each carrying potential therapeutic benefits. These components, when combined with other natural products, could offer new therapeutic alternatives, but we need a broader cannabis education to know more.

The current focus on THC and CBD, fueled by media hype, overshadows the rich complexity and full therapeutic spectrum of the cannabis plant. Acknowledging this diversity is crucial for developing comprehensive treatment plans that leverage the entire plant's potential.

Myrcene is known for its sedative properties, making it ideal for sleep-inducing blends, while limonene offers a more uplifting and euphoric experience, often sought after for its mood-enhancing effects. Additionally, the versatility of cannabis genetics allows for cultivation in a variety of broad spectrum flavors and aromas ranging from earthy and herbal to sweet and citrusy, catering to individual preferences and therapeutic needs.

This diversity not only enriches the user experience but also broadens the scope of personalized medicine, enabling patients to find the precise combination that works best for their specific conditions and lifestyles.

These specialized strains have led to the development of various products, including tinctures and oils, tailored for therapeutic use.

In regions where it's legal, individuals often craft their tinctures, and numerous NGOs and caregiver clubs can guide you to create these preparations safely at home. Specialized infusers, no bigger than a crock pot, can facilitate the tincture-making process as well. For those interested in exploring homemade tinctures, reaching out to these organizations can offer valuable resources and ensure the final product is free from contaminants.

Sacks also touched on the critical role of patient education in cannabis use, particularly regarding the entourage effect of cannabinoids (see Chapter 1) and terpenes in symptom management and regarding reducing dependence on traditional pharmaceuticals such as opioids and hypnotics.

Traditional medications such as opioids and hypnotics often come with significant side effects, including addiction, gastrointestinal issues, and cognitive impairment, posing substantial risks, especially to older patients.

In contrast, cannabis offers a safer alternative with fewer and more manageable side effects, providing a promising path towards reducing dependency on these potent drugs and enhancing quality of life.

Guidelines for different delivery methods

Each delivery method has different reaction times, and hardly any are instantaneous. Because of the varied delayed onset times, it can be tempting to believe it's "not working" and take another puff or eat another half of a brownie. But remember, go slow. Be patient.

For newcomers to smoking or vaporization, start with one inhalation and wait ten minutes before assessing effects to prevent overconsumption and euphoria. The medication enters the bloodstream rapidly, with effects felt within 60 to 90 seconds, peaking at around 15 minutes. The duration of these effects in the body is approximately 2 to 3 hours. However, if you over consume, it may take 2 to 3 hours to experience relaxation.

With tinctures or sublingual products, you will feel the effects after 15 to 30 minutes. Wait another 30 minutes after that to see how you feel before you take a higher dose. If it's your first time trying that product, it is going to stay in the body for about 4 to 6 hours or 6 to 8 hours.

Edible products, such as gummies, capsules, and cookies, pose unique challenges. The size of these products does not necessarily dictate their strength, making it essential to understand dosing. Edibles take the longest to take effect, typically 1 to 3 hours, but factors like the composition of recent meals can influence absorption, with fatty meals potentially enhancing the absorption of cannabinoids.

It might be tempting to over consume edibles due to their significant delayed onset. This can lead individuals to mistakenly take more before feeling any effects. Edibles also have a longer duration of action, staying in the body for 8 to 10 hours or 6 to 8 hours, depending on one's metabolism. "For newcomers or those unprepared for such long-lasting effects, this can lead to discomfort and anxiety," Dr. Charles warns.

Methods of cannabis delivery

The array of methods for cannabis use, from inhalation to edibles, offers varied implications for patient care, underlining the importance of a deep understanding of the endocannabinoid system.

Type	Method	Description	Pros	Cons
Smoking	Joints and blunts	Cannabis rolled in papers or tobacco leaves.	Simple to roll, convenient.	Odor, lung damage, shorter effects.
	Pipes	Handheld devices for quick smoking.	Easy to use, portable.	Lung damage, strong odor.
	Bongs and water pipes	Water-filtered pipes for smoother smoke.	A smoother hit, rapid onset.	Bulky, requires maintenance, lingering odor.
	Hookahs	Multi-stemmed pipes adapted for cannabis.	Social, allows group use.	Difficult to set up, bulky, odor.
	Homemade devices	DIY devices like gravity bongs.	Innovative, low-cost.	Potential health hazards, inefficiency.
Vaporizing	Portable vaporizers	Handheld vaporizers for flowers or concentrates.	Discreet, less lung damage.	Initial cost, learning curve.

(Continued)

Type	Method	Description	Pros	Cons
	Desktop vaporizers	Larger units with more control options.	Precise temperature control, potent hits.	Expensive, not portable, and require maintenance.
	Vape pens	Battery-powered pens with pre-filled cartridges.	Portable, discreet, easy to use.	Potential additive concerns, limited customization.
Edibles	Baked goods	Cannabis-infused baked products like brownies.	Long-lasting effects, discreet.	Delayed onset, can be too potent.
	Candies and gummies	Infused sweets like candies and gummies.	Easy to dose, long-lasting.	Delayed onset, potential overconsumption.
	Beverages	Cannabis-infused drinks like teas or sodas.	Discreet, long-lasting effects.	Difficult dosing, slower onset.
	Savory foods	Infused snacks or culinary items.	Variety, discreet, flavorful.	Difficult to dose, slower onset.
Tinctures	Sublingual tinctures	Cannabis extracts are applied under the tongue.	Fast onset, precise dosing.	Taste can be unpleasant, and less potent.
	Capsules and pills	Cannabis oil in pill form for oral ingestion.	Easy to dose, discreet, familiar form.	Slow onset, may have inconsistent effects.
	Sprays	Cannabis sprays are administered orally.	Discreet, rapid onset.	Limited availability, the taste may be unpleasant.

Type	Method	Description	Pros	Cons
Topicals	Creams and lotions	Cannabis-infused skincare products for localized use.	Non-psychoactive, easy to apply.	Limited effect, may not work for everyone.
	Transdermal patches	Patches delivering cannabinoids through the skin.	Discreet, long-lasting, potent.	Limited availability, can be expensive.
Concentrates (can also be consumed through vaping, adding to food or drinks and using in edibles)	Dabbing	Inhaling vapor from heated cannabis extracts. (hash, resin, live resin, and other form factors)	Rapid onset, very potent.	Requires equipment, which may be over-whelming.
Suppositories	Rectal suppositories	Rectally administered cannabis for systemic relief.	Avoids GI tract, and rapid absorption.	Less common, can be invasive.
	Vaginal suppositories	Vaginally administered for localized and systemic relief.	Targeted relief, avoids the GI tract.	Less common, can be invasive.
Inhalers	Metered-dose inhalers	Cannabis in metered-dose inhalers for precise dosing.	Precise dose, rapid onset.	Limited avail-ability, can cause throat irritation.
Ingestible oils	Oral intake (in drops or similar format)	Highly concentrated cannabis oil for oral ingestion.	Highly potent, long-lasting.	Strong flavor, difficult to dose.

However, as these methods gain popularity, be careful of sub-standard products. They pose significant dangers, especially to those with neurological conditions or compromised immune systems. Any cannabis product you consider using should adhere to stringent quality and safety standards to avoid the risks of heavy metals, pesticides, and fungal toxins.

When considering various cannabis consumption methods, know their key precautions and advantages. For instance, inhalation methods, such as vaping, offer immediate relief and dosage control, making them suitable for acute symptoms like pain or nausea, but may not be ideal for individuals with respiratory issues.

Topicals, on the other hand, can offer localized relief from pain and inflammation without psychoactive effects, representing a safe alternative for elderly patients or those new to cannabis.

Edibles provide a discreet and controlled dosage option, beneficial for those requiring long-lasting relief without the risks associated with smoking, yet they require careful dosing due to delayed onset of effects.

Challenges of edible consumption

Understanding dosing with edibles is crucial but challenging, in part due to the lack of regulation. For instance, a seemingly small product like a cookie may contain more THC and CBD than a larger gummy, leading to unpredictable effects.

While cannabis is generally safe, acknowledging and managing potential side effects is essential. To address and reverse the effects of excessive THC consumption, Dr. Charles recommends considering CBD. CBD competes for the same receptors as THC but acts differently. While THC activates the receptor, CBD sits on it, effectively blocking it and turning it off. This action induces the production of natural cannabinoids in the body. If you've consumed too much THC, taking higher doses of CBD can compete for those receptors, reducing the activation of THC. This competition helps bring you back to a more comfortable state.

The availability of different product ratios, especially in medical markets, further supports tailored cannabis experiences. Products with balanced THC and CBD ratios, such as 1:1 or 1:20, provide pain relief without the heavy euphoria associated with THC.

Set and setting

There are strategies to mitigate potential side effects, such as hydration, rest, and preparing your environment beforehand. Consuming cannabis in an environment with loud noises, unfamiliar faces, bright lights, and a fast-paced atmosphere can lead to a vastly more negative experience compared to a more comfortable setting such as relaxing on your couch at home, or in a familiar public space or out in nature with your friends.

Listen to your body and communicate any adverse reactions to your healthcare provider to ensure a responsive and personalized approach to cannabis treatment.

Warning: Who should not consume cannabis?

Dr. Peter Grinspoon discusses the risks of consuming cannabis, who should not consume it, and who should be careful:

> "There are certain populations that shouldn't use cannabis or should use it with extreme caution. You know teenagers, we're concerned about the effect of development on the teenage brain, particularly up until age 18."

He adds that teenagers should avoid cannabis unless facing severe medical conditions, such as terminal cancer. Also those individuals with a history of psychosis or those with a familial predisposition to psychotic disorders should be very wary of medical cannabis. While cannabis does not cause schizophrenia—a condition with stable incidence rates despite increased cannabis usage—it can precipitate its onset earlier in life. Dr. Grinspoon explains:

> "Cannabis doesn't cause schizophrenia . . . but it can precipitate it earlier, which is really bad . . . And schizophrenia can destabilize people with psychosis who have a predisposition to it."

Moreover, he points out that cannabis can exacerbate conditions like bipolar disorder, leading to manic episodes.

Pregnancy and breastfeeding present another area where the safety of cannabis use is not established, prompting caution. Dr. Grinspoon advises:

"We have no idea if it's safe or not in pregnancy or breastfeeding. There's no evidence that it is safe. As a primary care doctor, I'm really careful with everything during pregnancy and breastfeeding."

Addiction remains a contentious issue, and Dr. Grinspoon is critical of the inflated addiction rates often reported. He argues that the criteria used to define cannabis use disorder are influenced by outdated perspectives from the War on Drugs, leading to misleading statistics, and advocates for a more nuanced understanding of cannabis dependency:

"Now people do get addicted to cannabis. The rates of addiction have been wildly exaggerated because psychiatrists have these Drug War-informed definitions of cannabis use disorder."

He acknowledges that while withdrawal from cannabis can indeed affect mood, leading to irritability and sleep disturbances, these symptoms are less severe than those associated with harder substances. Dr. Grinspoon explains:

"You do have withdrawal symptoms from cannabis. You get grumpy, you can't sleep. That sucks. But it's not like you feel like you're going to die, like an opiate withdrawal."

Understanding individual tolerance

When considering cannabis as a therapeutic alternative, it's important to recognize that each individual's system is unique. This uniqueness translates into varying tolerance levels and responses to external interventions, including treatments aimed at regulating this system. Just as each person has a distinct set of life experiences and genetic makeup, so too does their endocannabinoid system present its specific baseline. Understanding and respecting this individual variability is key to effectively addressing and tuning each person's internal harmony to their optimal state.

For instance, 10mg of THC might surpass a person's tolerance level, while someone else, regardless of their size or age, might need 20mg to reach that point. In microdosing, smaller doses, typically ranging from two and a half to five milligrams, are administered gradually. The aim is to relieve pain or alleviate symptoms without crossing the threshold into euphoria.

Specific populations

When it comes to cannabis use, it's crucial to recognize that specific groups of people might have unique needs and benefits.

Dr. Genester Wilson-King, a renowned advocate, speaker, clinician, and educator in the fields of cannabis and hormone/wellness therapy, discusses how cannabis can be particularly effective for individuals going through menopause. It can help regulate mood swings and manage other symptoms associated with this natural phase of life.

"Cannabis is not going to replace or supplement the hormonal environment in your body. It won't cause you to have more estrogen or more progesterone or anything like that. It's not a substitute for hormonal therapy, but it can help some of the symptoms caused by hormonal imbalance."

Furthermore, Dr. Wilson-King elaborates on the broader benefits of cannabis, emphasizing its holistic impact:

"THC certainly can help with mood . . . the combination of THC and CBD, like the whole plant and the terpenes, all help with mood. Limonene is great for the treatment of depression. So the whole plant can help with depression, anxiety . . . various parts of the cannabis plant are very helpful in female conditions."

Meanwhile, Dr. Donald Abrams, a specialist in integrative medicine and cancer treatment at the UCSF Osher Center for Integrative Health, highlights the therapeutic potential of cannabis in alleviating common symptoms in HIV patients, such as nausea, pain, appetite loss, insomnia, anxiety, and depression. He emphasizes the importance of considering the whole plant and the synergistic "entourage effect" of its components.

Moreover, Dr. Abrams discusses his research on cannabis and the immune system in HIV patients:

"We did a very intensive study . . . comparing cannabis to dronabinol and a placebo, looking at the impact on the immune system and we found no detriment."

He notes an increase in lymphocyte numbers, crucial for HIV patients, highlighting the nuanced yet potentially beneficial role of cannabis in managing not just symptoms but also contributing positively to the immune system's functioning.

Dr. Paloma Lehfeldt, a lifelong cannabis advocate who serves as the director of Medical Education for Vireo Health, and with more than 10 years of experience in psychiatric research, adds:

"In medicine, we always weigh risks against benefits, and we discuss contraindications, which identify individuals who should avoid or use caution with certain substances. These are divided into relative and absolute contraindications. Absolute contraindications include a history of psychosis or bipolar I disorder, particularly due to the manic phase, because THC can exacerbate these conditions."

Additionally, individuals with a first-degree relative with these disorders should also avoid cannabis, as it can potentially unmask these symptoms.

These warnings extend to people with a history of addiction or adverse reactions to cannabis, those with severe cardiovascular conditions like myocardial infarction or certain arrhythmias since THC can worsen these issues, and pregnant or lactating women. Dr. Lehfeldt advises:

"The medical consensus, based on the current understanding that cannabis crosses the placenta and can affect the fetus, advises against the use of cannabis in these groups until more research is available. In every aspect of the conversation about cannabis, the need for more research is a constant theme."

Understanding cannabis interactions with other medications is vital. Dr. Grinspoon and Dr. Kogan emphasize the importance of consulting with healthcare providers to manage these interactions effectively, particularly in populations like older adults or those with complex medical conditions. Dr. Kogan notes:

"I quickly found from my patients, mostly in combination with literature, of course, is that for older adults, it became such a valuable tool and such a powerful tool and so safe that I never looked back . . . Cannabis now is a first or second line for at least half a dozen conditions."

Conclusion

In this chapter, we've explored the nuanced landscape of medical cannabis, guided by the expertise of Dr. Mikhail Kogan, Cheri Sacks, Dr. Duclas Charles, and other health professionals. Their collective insights illuminate the path towards safely integrating cannabis into medical treatment, especially for older adults and individuals seeking alternatives to conventional medications. Emphasizing patient-centric approaches, personalized healthcare plans, and the importance of precise dosing, these professionals underscore the therapeutic potential of cannabis when used responsibly.

We've learned about the "start low and go slow" principle, the significance of understanding individual tolerance, and the importance of choosing the correct delivery method to maximize benefits while minimizing risks. The chapter also highlighted the critical role of patient education in navigating the complexities of cannabis use, ensuring patients are well-informed about their treatments.

Special attention was given to the potential interactions between cannabis and other medications, urging a collaborative effort between patients and healthcare providers to manage these interactions effectively. This is particularly important for older adults and those with complex medical conditions, where the goal is not only symptom management but also enhancing the overall quality of life.

As we conclude, it's clear that the evolving landscape of medical cannabis offers promising avenues for treatment, backed by a growing body of research and clinical experience. The insights shared in this chapter serve as a valuable resource for patients and practitioners alike, advocating for a well-informed, cautious approach to cannabis use in medical practice. This forward-looking perspective encourages embracing the therapeutic benefits of cannabis while navigating its challenges with care and expertise, signaling a hopeful direction for the future of personalized medicine.

12

Navigating legalities and ethics of medical cannabis use

This chapter bridges the gap between the burgeoning promise of cannabis in healthcare and the complex realities of its application in modern medicine.

With contributions from leading experts in the field—Drs. Marion McNabb, Duclas Charles, Marcelo Morante, Paloma Lehfeldt, and Monica Werkheiser—we aim to offer a panoramic view of the nuanced dilemmas healthcare providers, patients, and policymakers face in navigating the medical cannabis ecosystem.

Our exploration begins with an in-depth look at the ethical considerations surrounding the prescription of medical marijuana, where medical efficacy meets regulatory scrutiny, and patient care intersects with evolving evidence.

As we do so, we invite you to consider the balance between potential benefits and the responsibilities incumbent upon prescribing practitioners in ensuring patient safety.

On the other hand, the legal labyrinth of medical cannabis use, marked by the dichotomy between state-level acceptance and federal prohibition, presents its own set of hurdles for patients, healthcare providers, and legal experts alike.

These pages aim to shed light on these legal intricacies, offering insights into how legal challenges shape access to treatment, research endeavors, and the responsibilities of consumers within the medical cannabis landscape. Likewise, the paramount importance of patient rights and access to treatment will emerge as a central theme.

As we conclude the exploration of these broader themes, we underscore the importance of equipping both providers and patients with the knowledge necessary for informed decision-making. This sets the stage for a deep dive into the ethical dilemmas faced by healthcare providers, where the responsibility to the patient, adherence to legal frameworks, and the leveraging of emerging evidence are delicately balanced.

The following section picks up this thread by focusing on the concrete ethical quandaries encountered by medical professionals in the act of prescribing cannabis.

As we delve into these ethical considerations, we continue to draw upon the invaluable insights of our contributors, whose experiences and expertise illuminate the path through this challenging yet crucial aspect of medical cannabis use.

Ethical considerations in prescribing cannabis

While understanding the ethical landscape of prescribing medical cannabis, healthcare providers and caretakers grapple with a complex array of considerations that balance patient care, legal regulations, and emerging evidence on efficacy and safety.

Navigating ethical boundaries as healthcare professionals

Dr. Duclas Charles' perspective as a pharmacist and cannabis expert sheds light on the nuanced ethical considerations in prescribing cannabis:

> "As a pharmacist, I must be cautious in stating categorically that cannabis is beneficial for specific conditions without FDA approval. My professional stance allows me to reference patient testimonials rather than make direct claims. This approach aligns with current regulations."

However, while the primary approach is to prescribe cannabis for conditions with a substantial evidence base, anecdotal and empirical evidence from patients, caretakers, and healthcare providers suggest that the therapeutic effects of cannabis extend well beyond these documented uses.

The broad therapeutic spectrum of cannabis: Challenges in standardizing treatment

As it stands, there is a body of empirical evidence which points to the potential of cannabis to treat a wider array of pathologies than commonly recognized, challenging the conventional boundaries of medical cannabis application.

The exploration into the medicinal potential of cannabis is not just about THC and CBD; rare cannabinoids, flavonoids, and terpenes play significant roles, yet their effects remain largely under-researched. These compounds contribute to the therapeutic landscape of cannabis in ways we are only beginning to understand, a fact that suggests a rich field of study for future research.

Adding to the complexity is the endocannabinoid system, a sophisticated network that maintains bodily homeostasis and influences numerous physiological processes. The ECS's complexity, alongside the entourage effect—whereby the therapeutic benefits of the whole cannabis plant exceed the sum of its parts—stands in contrast to the linear logic of traditional medicine, which typically prescribes a specific treatment for specific symptoms and awaits a predictable response. For these reasons, the prescription of cannabis remains a nuanced and intricate process.

The therapeutic potential of cannabis, therefore, cannot be fully realized through a linear approach; instead, it requires a comprehensive understanding of its complex interactions within the body, highlighting the need for further research and a more sophisticated framework for its clinical application.

Risks and modalities of consumption

The use of cannabis also carries risks, particularly regarding mental health. Evidence links it to an increased incidence of anxiety in a dose-dependent manner, especially for teenagers under the age of 18 and those with a history or family history of mental health disorders.

Furthermore, the modalities of cannabis consumption, from smoking and edibles to tinctures and topicals, introduce additional variables in assessing both therapeutic outcomes and potential risks.

Navigating ethical prescribing amid legal discrepancies

Ethical prescribing involves guiding patients towards safe consumption methods, as well as considering the potency and the balance of THC and CBD, which can influence both efficacy and side effects. The contested status of cannabis in many societies, combined with the legal discrepancies between state and federal regulations, adds another layer of ethical complexity, particularly in navigating patient education, shared decision-making, and the provider's ongoing clinical education to stay abreast of the evolving landscape.

Given these considerations, it's clear that the ethical recommendation of medical cannabis is not just about legality or patient demand, but requires a nuanced understanding of an individual's condition, the potential benefits and risks of cannabis use, and the broader social and legal context.

Patient rights and access to treatment

Many healthcare providers are restricted from becoming licensed recommenders of cannabis because most operate outside the conventional healthcare system. As Dr. McNabb explains:

> "I wouldn't go to my primary care provider to ask for a medical cannabis consultation because, often, ongoing healthcare systems do not permit their physicians or nurses to become licensed recommenders of medical cannabis."

This limitation results in a disconnect between patients and their usual healthcare providers, leading to the emergence of specialty clinics. This can be majorly inconvenient for patients who must seek medical cannabis certification outside their usual healthcare routine, often incurring additional costs. Dr. McNabb adds:

> "It's often difficult for patients to discuss their cannabis use with their regular healthcare providers. The challenge extends to obtaining a certification card and integrating that with one's standard care, especially in ensuring that cannabis use does not adversely interact with other medications. This is particularly problematic when primary care providers are not fully informed about cannabis's medical benefits and risks."

For patients in recovery from opioid addiction, many recovery programs test for cannabis use and may expel participants if cannabis is detected.

All this emphasizes the necessity of dismantling barriers to access and fostering an environment where patients can explore cannabis as a treatment option under the guidance of knowledgeable healthcare providers. In addition, Dr. Morante pointed to the transformative impact of cannabis legalization in Argentina on patient access, especially for those suffering from chronic pain and neurological conditions.

In line with Dr. Morante, Dr. Werkheiser notes the importance of dismantling barriers for patients, especially those in conservative or underserved areas.

Ethical implications of home cultivation

The responsibility for ethical implications does not fall solely on healthcare providers. Consumers and growers in the medical cannabis landscape must also include the ethical consideration of sourcing and production. While not everyone can cultivate their cannabis, in regions where it is legal, home cultivation emerges as a viable alternative to ensure traceability and purity from pesticides and heavy metals.

This self-sufficiency not only provides consumers with a direct line to their medicine, ensuring its cleanliness and efficacy, but also empowers them with the knowledge and skills to produce various forms of cannabis treatments, such as oils and ointments, tailored to their specific needs.

Moreover, the act of growing cannabis at home transcends the practical benefits of having a steady supply of medication; it encompasses the therapeutic benefits of gardening itself, which many find to be a tranquil and rewarding endeavor.

This holistic approach to wellness—combining the physical benefits of marijuana with the mental health benefits of gardening—presents an integrative model of health that aligns with the ethos of patient empowerment and self-care.

Moreover, the accessibility of cultivation kits and the wealth of information available online make this a feasible option for many; a stark contrast to barriers to access that can exist in traditional healthcare settings.

According to Dr. Morante, promoting the idea of home cultivation within legal boundaries is not about circumventing medical advice or the healthcare system. Rather, "it's about expanding the concept of treatment to include patient-led initiatives and alternative therapies that complement conventional medical care."

Thus, teaching and encouraging patients to grow their own medicine where legally permissible is an ethical stance rooted in advocating for patient autonomy, self-reliance, and the right to holistic health. It underscores a commitment to patient education and empowerment, emphasizing the value of understanding and taking control of one's treatment path.

This perspective posed by Dr. Morante challenges the notion that access to cannabis—and by extension, relief from various conditions—should solely rely on the medical system and its gatekeepers. By advocating for home cultivation as a supplement to professional medical advice, Dr. Morante addresses broader issues of accessibility, affordability, and personal agency in healthcare.

The democratization of access to cannabis treatment reveals the importance of making therapeutic options available beyond the confines of traditional medical consultations. This inclusivity ensures that individuals willing to dedicate time and effort to their health can also explore the benefits of cannabis.

For tips on how to get started growing your own cannabis, see Appendix A and Appendix B.

Ethical implications of cannabis research

On a similar note, the ethical landscape of cannabis research is marked by a series of complex challenges and dilemmas, reflecting the tension between societal perceptions, legal constraints, capitalistic drivers, and the scientific pursuit of knowledge.

Research needs to thoroughly examine both the therapeutic applications and potential risks associated with cannabis use. Not many published studies to date transcend the binary of beneficial versus harmful effects. The current research environment, influenced by both market demands and patient advocacy, faces the challenge of aligning commercial interests with genuine medical needs.

The question arises: Is the direction of cannabis research being driven more by market opportunities or by the voices of patients and the medical community? This dilemma is crucial, as it impacts the types of studies funded and the areas of research prioritized.

Dr. Morante's critique of the existing bias in research funding towards highlighting the negative effects of cannabis calls for a more equitable approach to research.

Moreover, the dominance of certain cannabis strains and genetic pools, tailored for specific market-oriented products, further complicates the landscape, raising questions about the breadth and depth of research into the plant's full spectrum of applications.

The challenges extend to the international and national legal frameworks that currently inhibit cannabis research. Restrictive treaties and laws significantly limit the available budget for comprehensive studies, particularly those exploring the endocannabinoid system and the entourage effect.

The lack of funding from public universities and national research programs for cannabis studies stifles the advancement of knowledge in this critical area, leaving significant gaps in our understanding of cannabis's mechanisms and effects.

The scarcity of allocated funds for cannabis research from reputable institutions points to a systemic issue within the scientific and medical research communities and is a reflection of a hesitancy to fully embrace cannabis studies due to legal and societal pressures.

Besides, the legal ambiguity surrounding cannabis's status in various regions presents a significant ethical dilemma, compounded by the overarching need for comprehensive education within the healthcare sector.

Legal challenges and consumer responsibilities

The intricate legal landscape surrounding medical cannabis presents a significant challenge for companies and healthcare providers operating within an environment where cannabis remains federally illegal.

In the USA, this disparity between state legalization and federal prohibition exposes businesses to considerable legal risks, including potential lawsuits that could jeopardize their financial stability and operational viability.

Companies, regardless of size, face the daunting prospect of bankruptcy should they find themselves embroiled in legal battles, a situation exacerbated by the cannabis industry's issues with traceability. The lack of federal banking access for cannabis businesses hinders their ability to manage finances, tax deductions, and access to financing, placing an additional strain on operational sustainability—at the time of the writing of this book, cannabis hadn't been rescheduled under federal law; if rescheduling were to go through, some of these barriers could be eliminated.

Besides, the absence of a federally sanctioned control system complicates the verification of product origins and testing and limits the availability of legally compliant products. Thus, ensuring product quality and consumer safety proves to be a challenge, as regulated markets and rigorous lab testing are not universal.

For providers, the discrepancies between federal and state laws create a complex scenario. They must navigate the legal intricacies of prescribing cannabis, often without the support of healthcare programs to cover the plant as a medicine. This coverage gap, combined with a general lack of awareness among medical providers about the full spectrum of cannabis's therapeutic possibilities, greatly restricts patient access to potentially beneficial treatments.

However, the potential rescheduling of cannabis could alleviate many of these concerns, by redefining its legal status to reflect a more nuanced understanding of its risks relative to substances like cocaine and heroin. Such a shift could pave the way for integrated supply chains, broader market access, and a reduction in the legal risks currently stifling industry growth.

Until such changes are implemented, the cannabis industry and its stakeholders must navigate a precarious legal environment, marked by significant risks that can deter investment, innovation, and the expansion of therapeutic options for patients.

Trustworthy products and safety concerns

In discussing ethical considerations in cannabis treatment, Dr. Morante explains the ethical responsibility of healthcare providers to explore all therapeutic options, including cannabis, for conditions lacking effective treatments. By educating patients and carefully considering cannabis as part of a comprehensive treatment plan, providers can find a balance between potential benefits and ethical obligations.

The therapeutic use of cannabis can bring ethical results. In clinical settings, he explains, patients using cannabis can reduce their reliance on opioids and other medications with known long-term adverse effects, particularly in managing chronic diseases to enhance the quality of life and expand therapeutic options for conditions like pain.

However, cannabis also poses a challenge for both the patient and the scientific community in which the person is embedded. Although cannabis still lacks the appropriate regulatory frameworks, new research and discoveries in the field of integrative medicine allow medical professionals and caretakers to evaluate the use of traditional treatments.

The ethical question arises from the balance between offering relief through the therapeutic use of marijuana and facing the challenges posed by the current lack of regulatory frameworks. Besides, all this must include the consideration of a fundamental ethical principle in medicine: to do no harm.

By considering cannabis as a treatment option, healthcare providers are weighing the potential to reduce harm from conventional treatments against the need for rigorous, evidence-based practice in an area still emerging from regulatory and scientific uncertainty.

Hence, the ethical dilemma lies in making informed decisions that prioritize patient welfare while acknowledging the evolving understanding of cannabis's role in medical treatment.

Conclusion

All in all, the journey ahead is both promising and fraught with challenges, particularly regarding the potential health benefits of cannabis and the complex ethical, legal, and social considerations that accompany its integration into medical practice. The insights from leading experts form a collective call to action: to face these complexities with informed compassion, rigorous research, and unwavering advocacy.

The future of medical cannabis hinges on our ability to balance these considerations, forging a path that respects patient autonomy, ensures equitable access, and upholds the highest standards of care. As we look forward, several key themes emerge as guideposts for this journey:

- **Empowering patients and providers**: Education is paramount. Both patients and healthcare providers need comprehensive, evidence-based information to make informed decisions about cannabis use. This includes understanding the nuances of cannabis pharmacology, the implications of various administration methods, and the legal landscape surrounding cannabis prescription and use.
- **Advancing research**: The call for more research is a clarion one. Future breakthroughs in cannabis medicine depend on rigorous, well-funded studies that explore the full spectrum of cannabis's therapeutic potential, including its risks and benefits. This research must also extend to understanding the best practices for integrating cannabis into holistic treatment plans.
- **Navigating legal challenges**: Legal reform is critical to the future of medical cannabis. Changing federal classification, harmonizing state and federal laws, and establishing clear, consistent regulations will be crucial in ensuring safe, legal access to marijuana for therapeutic use. These changes will also facilitate research and allow healthcare providers to incorporate cannabis into their practice without fear of legal repercussions.
- **Ethical prescribing practices**: As cannabis becomes more integrated into medical treatment, ethical considerations around prescribing practices will become increasingly important. Providers will need to balance the desire to alleviate suffering with the need to ensure patient safety, considering the complex interplay of factors such as potential side effects, interactions with other medications, and the risk of dependency.

- **Social equity and access**: Ensuring equitable access to medical cannabis is a moral imperative. Future policies must address the disparities in cannabis access and affordability, particularly for marginalized communities disproportionately impacted by previous drug policies. This includes considering models for nonprofit distribution, subsidies for low-income patients, and community-based education initiatives.
- **Patient-centered care**: Ultimately, the future of medical cannabis must be rooted in a patient-centered approach. This means respecting patient autonomy, prioritizing their well-being, and recognizing the therapeutic potential of marijuana as part of a comprehensive care strategy. It also means advocating for policies and practices that support patient access to cannabis medicine, including the right to grow this plant for personal use where legally permissible.

13

The future of medical cannabis

This chapter explores the evolution of medical cannabis, highlighting its journey from an ancient medicine to future treatments, driven by technological advancements and changing
societal attitudes. As we stand on the brink of a new era in healthcare, cannabis emerges as a key player in the movement towards
more personalized and holistic treatments.

This chapter delves into the economic, regulatory, and technological challenges and opportunities facing medical cannabis.
We explore the pivotal role of digital health technologies in
enhancing patient care, highlighted by Cheri Sacks' insights into
leveraging these tools for personalized cannabis treatment plans.
Sacks' experience underlines the impact of digital innovations
in tracking dosages, symptoms, and patient responses, offering a
more nuanced approach to cannabis-based therapy.

We also explore the burgeoning interest in minor cannabinoids
such as CBN, CBG, and CBC, and their distinct therapeutic benefits. The advent of synthetic cannabinoid production, offering precision and consistency, marks a significant leap towards integrating
cannabis more fully into medical practice and daily life.

Nanotechnology, a pivotal innovation in the design of cannabis-based therapies, manipulates substances at the molecular
level to enhance the delivery and efficacy of cannabinoids. This
technology significantly improves the bioavailability of cannabinoids, ensuring quicker absorption into the body's system and
optimizing therapeutic effects.

Through the microscopic precision of nanotechnology, cannabinoids can be engineered for more effective interaction with
the body's endocannabinoid system, paving the way for advancements in personalized medicine and patient care.

Amid these advancements, we confront the pressing need
for legal and regulatory reform to facilitate research and ensure

equitable access to cannabis treatments. The chapter argues for a reevaluation of cannabis's classification, emphasizing the potential for more structured and reliable therapeutic applications.

As we envision the future, we see a healthcare landscape where cannabis is not only accepted but integral to personalized medicine. This future is characterized by a synergy between technology and therapy, where digital health innovations, legal reforms, and a deeper understanding of cannabis's potential work together to offer tailored, effective treatments.

Chapter 13 serves as a forward-looking discussion on how the evolving landscape of medical cannabis can shape a more inclusive, innovative, and patient-centric healthcare system.

The dawn of a new era: From ancient remedy to modern marvel

The cannabis narrative is richly interwoven with human history, reflecting a dynamic interplay of economic, political, and social forces. In this modern age, cannabis stands at the forefront of medical innovation, propelled by a growing openness to its therapeutic possibilities. This resurgence is supported by the plant's regulatory and application advances in healthcare, signaling a shift towards more holistic and alternative health responses.

Modern resurgence in medical cannabis

The tradition of home cultivation, a practice with centuries-old roots, exemplifies cannabis's integral role in integrative medicine and alternative therapies. Accessibility to home cultivation, combined with an abundance of health-focused cultivation techniques, heralds cannabis as a formidable ally in the quest for holistic well-being. Yet, this path towards universal medicinal access encounters significant regulatory hurdles.

Economic and regulatory barriers to access

Regulations, while crucial for safety and efficacy, often impose barriers that limit access, particularly for those most in need. At the heart of the regulatory debate is the federal government's role in shaping cannabis's future. The plant's unique nature, especially concerning the endocannabinoid system and the entourage effect, challenges the conventional frameworks of pharmaceutical standardization. The ECS's complexity and individual variability, coupled with the synergistic potential of cannabis's phytochemicals, defy simple standardization, thus delaying the development of regulations.

This nuanced understanding paves the way for personalized and effective medical treatments, recognizing the plant's biochemistry and supporting traditional cultivation practices. As cannabis transitions from a historic remedy to a more widely accepted form of treatment, we are ushered into a new era of health and healing, marked by an evolving vision of cannabis fully integrated into therapeutic practices.

The narrative of cannabis is not just a reflection of its past but a projection towards its future, particularly at the intersection with digital health technologies.

As we delve into the next section, the focus shifts to these groundbreaking frontiers, where digital tools and technologies promise to enhance the personalization and efficacy of cannabis-based treatments.

Innovation's bloom: Technological advances in the cannabis industry

Leveraging her Silicon Valley background, in the following section registered nurse Cheri Sacks reveals the critical impact of digital health technologies in transforming cannabis treatment plans, especially for individuals grappling with chronic conditions. With her profound expertise in medical cannabis, behavior change, and managing chronic conditions, Sacks excels in devising personalized, cannabis health strategies with the assistance of digital technologies.

The role of digital health technologies in personalized care

The advent of digital health tools, including mobile apps for dosing and response tracking, marks a significant leap in personalizing healthcare. These innovations provide a granular understanding of individual responses to cannabis treatments, enabling real-time adjustments that refine therapeutic outcomes. Sacks explains:

> "Digital health technologies and medicinal cannabis are tools in our toolbox that can work well together. The more tools we have to support people, the more likely someone is to find one that works for them."

Moreover, a synergistic approach melds these technologies with established healthcare practices to cater to the unique medical histories, current medications, and cannabis experiences of individuals.

Journaling apps can facilitate detailed documentation of product effects on symptoms, thus enhancing pattern recognition and response management. In all, these digital technologies can educate and empower patients, challenging the stigmas surrounding cannabis use and ensuring a well-informed patient community.

Looking ahead, Sacks envisions a future where digital health technologies are integral to managing chronic conditions, predicting the development of innovative tools for virtual check-ins and precise dosing measurements. This perspective landscape promises a dynamic framework for cannabis therapy, optimizing patient outcomes through the convergence of digital health and medicinal marijuana, characterized by efficiency and personalization.

Unveiling the spectrum of minor cannabinoids

The cannabis industry is witnessing a significant shift towards the exploration of minor cannabinoids, such as CBN, CBG CBC, tetrahydrocannabivarin (THCV), and cannabidivarin (CBDV), each heralded for their distinct therapeutic benefits for different conditions and symptoms.

Such exploration also exemplifies the industry's commitment to leveraging cutting-edge technologies and scientific advancements.

CBN: A new frontier in sleep aid and beyond

CBN[105] has been particularly noted for its potential as a sleep aid,[106] and as a promising alternative for those seeking restful sleep without the psychotropic effects associated with THC. This compound is derived from the aging of THC: as THC degrades over time, especially under conditions of prolonged storage, high temperatures, and exposure to oxygen, CBN formation increases.

Currently, companies and consumers are progressively introducing CBN into the market in various forms such as tinctures, capsules, and gummies, often combined with melatonin and other sleep-enhancing aids.

Despite its growing popularity, the scientific foundation supporting CBN's efficacy as a sleep inducer primarily draws from anecdotal evidence and studies from the 1970s and 1980s, which suggest that while CBN alone may have minimal impact on sleep, its combination with THC could enhance sleepiness.[107]

However, the exploration of CBN's therapeutic potential doesn't stop at sleep; research hints at a broader spectrum of benefits:[108]

- pain management
- appetite stimulation
- immune support
- anti-inflammatory effects
- ADHD symptom management

Still, comprehensive research is needed to fully understand CBN's capabilities and its long-term effects.

Unlike its counterpart CBD, which has seen widespread study and FDA approval for specific medical uses, CBN's journey in scientific and medical communities is just beginning.[109] Nonetheless, the promise of CBN, especially when considered alongside other cannabinoids and terpenes,[110] suggests a synergistic potential that could redefine treatment paradigms across various conditions.

CBG and THCV: Targeting inflammation and appetite

CBG has captured interest for its anti-inflammatory and antibacterial properties, making it a candidate for treatments related to pain and swelling, especially post-exercise.

THCV stands out for its appetite-suppressing qualities, aligning with consumer interests in weight management and energy boost. Its stimulant-like effects make it a sought-after cannabinoid for those aiming to balance dietary intake and physical activity. Unlike its more famous counterparts such as THC, CBD, and CBN, THCV's effects and interactions present a novel area of exploration.[111]

In addition, THCV's role in appetite suppression diverges from the usual cannabis-induced "munchies," with most evidence rooted in animal studies suggesting that THCV may block the CB1 receptor, known to stimulate appetite. This blockade could potentially lead to reduced appetite and weight loss, as suggested by several animal studies.[112] However, human trials offer mixed results on THCV's efficacy as an appetite suppressant.[113] While THCV showed promise in reducing fasting plasma glucose and improving certain health markers, its impact on appetite and body weight remains unclear.

Despite this, preclinical research hints at THCV's potential across a spectrum of diseases and disorders, such as Parkinson's disease, psychosis, and pain, setting the stage for further investigation into this intriguing cannabinoid.

CBC: Enhancing mood and pain management

Currently, CBC is being explored for its mood-enhancing capabilities, potentially offering a new approach to wellness and mental health.

Discovered over 50 years ago, CBC does not bind well to CB1 receptors in the brain, which avoids psychotropic effects. However, it interacts with other body receptors involved in pain perception.[114] This interaction enhances the release of anandamide, a natural endocannabinoid, hinting at CBC's role in pain management and inflammation reduction.[115]

However, CBC's medicinal promise extends across various conditions, notably its potential in cancer therapy,[116] given its ability to maintain higher levels of anandamide in the bloodstream. Studies have highlighted its efficacy in inhibiting tumor growth and inflammation,[117] making it a candidate for chemo-preventive research.

Furthermore, CBC has demonstrated effectiveness in reducing pain and inflammation in osteoarthritis models, offering an alternative to traditional NSAIDs without the associated side effects.

With its impact on brain health, acne treatment,[118] and depression,[119] often enhanced by the entourage effect when combined with THC and CBD,[120] CBC could influence a vast therapeutic landscape. With ongoing research and evolving cannabis legislation, CBC's full spectrum of benefits presents a promising horizon for diversified cannabinoid-based therapies.

Revolutionizing cannabinoid production: The synthetic leap forward

The development of synthetic cannabinoids through innovative biosynthesis platforms represents a transformative leap in cannabinoid production. Techniques such as precision fermentation, utilizing yeast or sugar bases, enable the creation of pure, pharmaceutical-grade cannabinoids.

This method guarantees the purity and consistency necessary for pharmaceutical standards, making rare cannabinoids more accessible and aligning with the needs of patients requiring precise dosages and formulations.

For example, BayMedica's innovative biosynthesis platform highlights the feasibility of turning simple sugars into pure, pharmaceutical-grade cannabinoids, offering a sustainable and efficient alternative to plant-based extraction. This advancement not only holds the promise of making rare cannabinoids more accessible but also aligns with the pharmaceutical industry's standards for product safety and efficacy, essential for patients requiring precision in their treatments.

The future of cannabis lies not just in medicine but in the seamless integration of cannabinoids, terpenes, and flavonoids into daily life, including food and nutraceuticals. This holistic approach not only democratizes the benefits of cannabis but also opens the door to personalized health solutions.

With the capability to produce cannabinoids synthetically, companies can now infuse a wide range of products with precise doses of CBN, CBG, THCV, and more, catering to individual health needs and preferences.

This innovation dovetails with the concept of personalized medicine, offering targeted therapies and wellness products that adhere to the highest pharmaceutical standards, ensuring safety and efficacy for all users, including the immunosuppressed, elderly, and children.

This exploration of technological innovations in the cannabis industry serves as a prelude to the ensuing discussion on the shifting sands of public perception and the social impact of cannabis legalization.

As digital health technologies promise to refine and personalize cannabis therapies, they also play a crucial role in reshaping societal attitudes towards cannabis. The next section delves into the dynamic interplay between evolving public sentiment, legal landscapes, and the burgeoning role of cannabis in contemporary society.

The ripple effect: Evolving public perception and social impact

In the wake of advancements in digital health technologies within the cannabis sector, a parallel transformation is unfolding in the realm of public perception and social acceptance of cannabis.

This evolution is deeply influenced by myriad factors that signal a shift away from entrenched stigmas towards broader legalization and acceptance. Societal, political, economic, and ideological influences each play a pivotal role in reshaping the dialogue surrounding cannabis use and policy.

Crucially, generational shifts are at the heart of this changing landscape. Younger demographics, notably Millennials and Generation X, exhibit a markedly higher rate of support for cannabis legalization, a trend that reveals the impact of personal experience and cultural integration on public attitudes, a shift highlighted by Mosher and Atkins.[121]

Political ideologies and affiliations contribute to the discourse, with notable shifts among Republican Millennials towards legalization, suggesting a reevaluation of cannabis policies across traditional party lines. This evolution in political perspectives signifies a broader societal rethinking of cannabis, as we move towards more nuanced understandings beyond simplistic categorizations.

Social justice and legalization advocacy

This dialogue is further enriched by considerations of social justice, with the disproportionate impact of drug laws on minority communities fueling advocacy for legalization. This movement, as discussed by development scholars Tate, Taylor, and Sawyer,[122] aims to address systemic inequalities, exposing the critical social implications of cannabis legislation and the potential for reform to foster more equitable outcomes.

Empirical evidence and policy reform

Similarly, MacCoun and Reuter[123] examine the counterproductive outcomes of prohibition and call for alternative strategies that prioritize harm reduction and public health. The authors provide an analysis of how the USA should decide on the legal status of marijuana and draw upon data about the experiences of Western European nations with less punitive drug policies as well as analyses of America's experience with legal cocaine and heroin a century ago. Thus, their research shows that the choice about how to regulate drugs involves complicated tradeoffs and conflict among social groups.

Meanwhile, Brienen and Rosen[124] provide an analysis of the shift towards harm reduction and decriminalization in U.S. drug policy, accentuating the importance of evidence-based policy-making and the potential for policy reform to yield significant public health and economic benefits.

Towards a new paradigm in medical treatment

This exploration of the evolving public perception and social impact of cannabis sets the stage for the next discussion: the integration of medical cannabis into personalized medicine. As societal attitudes shift and the legal landscape evolves, the medical community stands on the brink of a paradigm shift.

The following section delves into how these changes pave the way for cannabis to play a pivotal role in tailored healthcare solutions, reflecting the broader implications of legalization, technological advancements, and changing societal norms on the future of medical treatment.

Personalized medicine

The narratives of professionals like Dr. Mikhail Kogan and Dr. Marcelo Morante are a testament to the necessity of moving beyond the conventional one-size-fits-all approach to embrace a more holistic, individualized, and patient-centric model of care.

The potential of medical cannabis to alleviate chronic pain, manage cancer symptoms, and address neurological disorders, among other conditions, proves its role as a valuable complement to traditional treatments. By integrating cannabis into a broader therapeutic strategy, healthcare can evolve to encompass a spectrum of options.

Acknowledging each patient's uniqueness is at the heart of personalized medicine. The stories of those treated by Dr. Kogan and Dr. Morante serve as an example of the individualized nature of medical care, where treatment plans are tailored to fit the specific physiological and psychological makeup of each person.

This approach is not merely about treating symptoms but about fostering an environment where wellness, balance, and harmony within the body are paramount. It reflects a future of healthcare that is not only reactive but also proactive, ensuring that every patient's journey through cannabis therapy is guided by knowledge, compassion, and precision.

This integration facilitates a comprehensive approach to health, emphasizing prevention, treatment, and the maintenance of optimal well-being. It challenges the medical community to expand its understanding and acceptance of cannabis, recognizing its potential to contribute significantly to personalized medicine.

As we delve into the future of medical cannabis, its role in personalized medicine becomes increasingly apparent, promising a new chapter in healthcare. This future, illuminated by the convergence of technological innovation, evolving societal attitudes, and the principles of personalized medicine, opens up a realm of possibilities for patient care.

Charting the course ahead: Rescheduling cannabis from Schedule I to Schedule III

In May of 2024 President Joe Biden announced his government would reclassify cannabis from a Schedule I to a Schedule III drug under federal law, marking a monumental shift in the landscape of medical cannabis. This move acknowledges the growing body of scientific evidence supporting the medicinal benefits of cannabis and represents a significant step towards rectifying long-standing inequities in drug policy.

Rescheduling cannabis to Schedule III will have profound implications for research, industry, and patient access. As a Schedule I substance, cannabis has been categorized alongside drugs considered to have no accepted medical use and a high potential for abuse, severely restricting research opportunities and imposing harsh legal penalties for possession and use. The reclassification to Schedule III, which denotes drugs with moderate to low potential for physical and psychological dependence and recognized medical uses, will dismantle many of these barriers.

For researchers, this reclassification will likely facilitate more comprehensive and rigorous scientific studies. Schedule I status has made it extremely difficult for scientists to obtain the necessary approvals and materials to conduct research on cannabis. Moving to Schedule III will streamline these processes, allowing for a more robust exploration of cannabis's therapeutic potentials and safety profiles. This, in turn, could lead to new cannabis-based treatments and a deeper understanding of its efficacy and mechanisms of action.

The cannabis industry will also experience significant changes. Schedule III status will alleviate some of the tax burdens imposed by the 280E provision of the Internal Revenue Code, which prohibits businesses dealing with Schedule I or II substances from deducting ordinary business expenses. This change will improve the financial viability of cannabis businesses, fostering growth and innovation within the industry. Additionally, it may encourage further investment and integration of cannabis into mainstream pharmaceutical and healthcare markets.

For patients, the reclassification promises improved access and affordability. With reduced legal barriers and increased research, patients will benefit from a greater variety of well-studied and regulated cannabis-based medications. Physicians, more confident in the legitimacy and safety of cannabis treatments, may be more likely to recommend them, leading to broader acceptance in the medical community. Furthermore, insurance companies might start covering cannabis-based treatments, making them more accessible to a wider population.

Future legal and ethical challenges

In contemplating the future of cannabis legalization, critical questions arise regarding equitable access and distribution. Will cannabis, once legalized, be accessible to all individuals, regardless of socioeconomic status, or will its availability be contingent upon purchasing power?

This pivotal inquiry underscores broader concerns regarding social justice and healthcare equity in the emerging landscape of legalized cannabis.

Moreover, as cannabis gains recognition for its therapeutic potential, questions emerge regarding its integration into educational curricula. Will schools and universities incorporate cannabis education to foster a comprehensive understanding of its nuanced applications and effects?

This consideration exhibits the necessity for informed discourse and evidence-based education to mitigate potential risks and maximize benefits associated with cannabis use.

Furthermore, the advent of synthetic cannabinoids introduces novel complexities to the cannabis market. Will these synthetic alternatives become the predominant means of accessing regulated cannabis, given their risk-free production methods?

Alternatively, will legalization extend to include provisions for home cultivation, communal growing initiatives akin to

Barcelona's cannabis clubs, or nonprofit organizations facilitating access?

The insights from Dr. Charles, combined with Dr. McNabb's expertise, paint a comprehensive picture of the future legal and ethical challenges in the field of medical cannabis. Their shared emphasis on education, regulatory clarity, and patient safety foregrounds the ongoing need for advocacy, research, and policy reform.

Reflecting on future challenges, Dr. Morante emphasizes the need for continuous dialogue and adaptation in the legal and ethical frameworks governing medical cannabis. He pointed to the dynamic nature of cannabis legislation in Argentina as a model for addressing future challenges, advocating for policies that are responsive to scientific advancements and societal needs.

Looking to the future, Dr. Werkheiser also expresses optimism about the integration of cannabis into mainstream healthcare, tempered by the recognition of ongoing legal and ethical challenges. She emphasized the importance of continued advocacy, research, and dialogue to ensure that cannabis's role in healthcare evolves in a manner that prioritizes patient well-being and safety.

Conclusion

The narrative of medical cannabis is at a pivotal juncture, reflecting a confluence of historical significance, evolving societal attitudes, and groundbreaking advancements in healthcare technology. In this context, the contributions from experts across the spectrum of healthcare, policy, and technology illuminate a path forward that is both innovative and reflective of the plant's storied past.

As we envision the future of medical cannabis, several key themes emerge as essential guideposts:

- **Embracing digital health technologies:** The integration of digital health technologies promises to revolutionize the personalization and effectiveness of cannabis-based treatments. Wearables, apps, and telehealth platforms offer new avenues for monitoring, education, and support, empowering patients and providers to tailor treatments precisely to individual needs and conditions. This technological synergy paves the way for a future where cannabis therapy is optimized through real-time data and insights, enhancing outcomes while maintaining a focus on patient safety and well-being.

- **Advocating for legal and regulatory reform**: The rescheduling of cannabis is a critical step towards unlocking its potential as a therapeutic agent. By reevaluating cannabis's classification and fostering a legal environment conducive to research and clinical application, we can dismantle barriers to access, facilitate rigorous scientific studies, and ensure that patients can benefit from cannabis's medicinal properties without navigating a maze of legal uncertainties. This shift requires a concerted effort from policymakers, healthcare professionals, and advocates to align cannabis regulation with contemporary scientific understanding and public health priorities.

- **Fostering education and breaking down stigmas**: Education plays a pivotal role in transforming perceptions and practices around medical marijuana. By disseminating evidence-based information, divulging patient success stories, and challenging outdated stigmas, we can cultivate a more informed and open-minded approach to cannabis in healthcare. This educational imperative extends to healthcare providers, patients, and the broader public, evidencing the need for ongoing dialogue, research dissemination, and community engagement.

- **Prioritizing equity and accessibility**: Ensuring equitable access to medical cannabis is fundamental to the ethos of healthcare. Addressing economic, regulatory, and social barriers to access is crucial for creating a healthcare landscape where all individuals, regardless of socioeconomic status or geographic location, can benefit from the plant's therapeutic potential. This includes advocating for affordable treatments, supporting home cultivation where legal, and developing policies that reflect a commitment to social justice and healthcare equity.

- **Exploring the full spectrum of cannabis medicine**: The future of medical cannabis lies in harnessing the full therapeutic spectrum of the plant, including minor cannabinoids, terpenes, and flavonoids. By embracing the complexity of the entourage effect and advancing research into these compounds, we can unlock new treatment avenues and refine our understanding of cannabis's role in healthcare. This exploration requires innovative research methodologies, cross-disciplinary collaboration, and a willingness to venture beyond conventional treatment paradigms.

14
Final words

Concluding the journey: Embracing cannabis as a pillar of modern medicine

This comprehensive guide on medical cannabis serves as a testament to the plant's intricate relationship with human health, offering a panoramic view of its historical journey, biological makeup, and therapeutic potential.

From its roots as an ancient remedy to its modern renaissance in medical science, cannabis emerges as a multifaceted ally in the quest for well-being, challenging longstanding stigmas and inspiring a new era of understanding and acceptance.

The exploration begins with a deep dive into cannabis's rich history and cultural impact, highlighting its evolution from traditional medicine to a subject of controversy and, finally, to a beacon of hope for many suffering from chronic conditions.

The guide further unfolds the complex biology of the cannabis plant, revealing the mechanisms through which it interacts with the human endocannabinoid system to offer relief and healing. This scientific inquiry extends into the realm of cultivation and extraction, emphasizing the importance of quality, safety, and innovation in harnessing cannabis's full therapeutic spectrum.

Through a lens of compassion and scientific rigor, the guide addresses cannabis's role in treating an array of conditions, from neurological disorders and mental health challenges to sleep disturbances and glaucoma.

Each chapter weaves together expert insights, clinical studies, and patient experiences, painting a picture of cannabis as a nuanced and potentially transformative element of medical treatment. Yet, it also calls attention to the need for careful consideration, personalized approaches, and continued research to fully understand and utilize cannabis's benefits.

The narrative underscores the significance of patient education, responsible use, and the harmonious integration of cannabis into healthcare practices. It advocates for a patient-centric approach, where informed decisions, precise dosing, and a deep respect for individual responses guide the therapeutic use of cannabis.

Moreover, it delves into the legal and ethical dimensions of medical cannabis, urging a collective effort towards regulatory reform, equitable access, and the dismantling of barriers to research and treatment.

Looking towards the horizon, the guide envisions a future where medical cannabis is seamlessly woven into the fabric of personalized and holistic healthcare. It champions the potential of technological advancements, the exploration of minor cannabinoids, and the vital role of advocacy in shaping policies that recognize and respect cannabis's medicinal value. This future is characterized by a healthcare landscape where cannabis is not only understood and accepted but also celebrated as a key component of comprehensive and compassionate care.

In sum, this guide serves as both a beacon of knowledge and a call to action, inviting readers to embark on a journey of discovery, advocacy, and hope. It challenges us to reimagine our relationship with cannabis, advocating for a world where its therapeutic potential is fully realized and integrated into the pursuit of health and happiness for all.

Appendix A
Cultivating cannabis outdoors

Cultivating cannabis at home is an accessible and rewarding endeavor, especially for those looking to grow their plants outdoors. With common supplies easily found at a supermarket, and a bit of know-how, anyone can start their cannabis cultivation journey. Here are some key supplies and tips to ensure a healthy growth cycle and bountiful harvest.

Key supplies for cannabis cultivation

1 **Soil**: Start with permeable soil that allows for good drainage and aeration. Cannabis plants thrive in soil that is neither too dense nor too compact, ensuring roots can breathe and expand freely.
2 **Worm castings**: During the vegetative phase, enriching your soil with worm castings can significantly benefit your cannabis plants with Nitrogen. These natural fertilizers are rich in nutrients and beneficial microorganisms, promoting healthy growth and robust development.
3 **Molasses (non-sulfured)**: In the flowering period, adding non-sulfured molasses to your watering mix can enhance bud development. Molasses acts as a carbohydrate supplement for the beneficial microbes in the soil, leading to improved nutrient uptake and healthier, more resinous flowers.

10 cultivation tips for success

1 **Understanding photoperiod vs. automatic plants**: Cannabis can be photoperiodic or auto-flowering. Photoperiod plants require specific light cycles to transition from vegetative growth to flowering, whereas auto-flowers will flower based on age, not light exposure. Tailor your care and attention to the type of plant you are growing.

2 **Lighting for outdoor cultivation**: Utilizing artificial lights outdoors can extend the vegetative phase by providing additional light during shorter days. This trick convinces the plant it's still summer, encouraging continued growth. Once artificial lighting is reduced, the plant perceives it as the approach of winter, triggering the flowering stage. This technique allows for flexibility in the growing schedule and can lead to larger yields.

3 **Seed selection**: For reputable seeds, consider purchasing from cannabis clubs in Europe, known for their quality genetics and as pioneers in the cannabis breeding industry since the 1970s and 1980s. These "souvenir" seeds are a reliable choice for growers seeking specific strain characteristics.

4 **Managing water and humidity**: Be cautious with watering: overwatering can lead to root issues and hinder plant health. To remove chlorine and ensure oxygen-rich water, let tap water sit in a bucket for a day or use a fish tank air pump to aerate the water for 24 hours before watering.

5 **Soil pH control**: Maintaining the correct pH level in your soil is crucial for nutrient uptake. For the vegetative stage, aim for a pH of 6.0-7.0, and for flowering, a slightly more acidic range of 6.0-6.5 is optimal.

6 **Use natural stimulants**: Such as lentil sprout juice, and beneficial fungi such as mycorrhizae, algae, Aloe Vera, and Lactobacillus for enhanced nutrient absorption.

7 **Growth and flowering time**: Cannabis growth stages are divided into vegetative and flowering phases. The vegetative stage can last 3-16 weeks when the plant develops its foliage and roots. The flowering stage follows, ranging from 8 to 11 weeks, during which the buds form and mature.

8 **Inspecting buds for harvest**: When the plant has matured, inspect the trichomes (the resinous glands) with a magnifier. The color shift from milky white to amber in these trichomes indicates readiness for harvest. This change signifies peak potency and is crucial for determining the best harvest time.

9 **Drying the buds**: Post-harvest, dry the buds in a dark place with low temperature and humidity, ensuring there's no direct wind flow and pets are kept away. It's vital to monitor

for any signs of mold, dark spots, or white cotton-like appearances on the buds. Hanging them upside down is a common practice during this stage.

10 **Curing for quality**: The final step, curing, involves placing the dried buds in airtight containers, opening them periodically to let air exchange, and checking for mold. Curing enhances the therapeutic effects and flavor of the cannabis by allowing a slow breakdown of chlorophyll and ensuring the trichomes mature properly. This process can significantly improve the quality and potency of the final product.

Appendix B
Indoor cannabis cultivation

Indoor cannabis cultivation offers growers control over environmental conditions, leading to potentially high-quality yields. However, it requires attention to detail and specific practices to ensure plant health and robust growth.

Here are essential tips for successful indoor cultivation:

1 **Cleanliness is crucial**: Maintain a sterile environment to prevent pests and diseases. Regularly clean your grow space, including floors, walls, and surfaces, to minimize the risk of mold and fungal infections such as botrytis, fusarium, oidium, and others that can harm both the plants and your health.

2 **Air filtration and ventilation**: Implement effective air filtration and ventilation systems to manage humidity and prevent the accumulation of mold spores and other airborne pathogens. Proper ventilation ensures fresh air circulation, preventing hot air pockets and maintaining a healthy environment for your plants.

3 **Watering and runoff control**: Monitor your watering practices closely. Ensure there's enough runoff to avoid nutrient buildup but not so much that it leads to nutrient loss. Overwatering can cause root rot, so balance is key. Using trays to catch runoff can help you manage water levels effectively.

4 **Wind and air movement**: Use fans to keep air moving within the grow space, but avoid directing airflow directly at plants to prevent wind stress. Consistent air movement helps regulate temperature and prevents hotspots, ensuring uniform plant growth.

5 **Optimal lighting**: Invest in quality lighting that covers the full spectrum needed for cannabis growth. LED lights are popular for their efficiency and lower heat output. Proper lighting is critical for photosynthesis and influences the vegetative and flowering stages.

6 **Temperature and humidity control**: Utilize air conditioning and dehumidifiers to keep the grow space within ideal temperature and humidity ranges. Ideal temperatures are generally between 70–80°F (21–25°C) during the day. Humidity levels should be adjusted according to the plant's growth stage, with lower humidity preferred during flowering.

7 **Pest control**: Be proactive in pest management. Regularly inspect plants for signs of infestation and employ organic pest control methods when possible. Keeping the grow area clean and monitoring plant health can prevent major outbreaks.

8 **Quality genetics and natural inputs**: Start with high-quality seeds or clones and use the same organic fertilizers and rooting supplements recommended for outdoor cultivation. Good genetics lay the foundation for vigorous growth and potent yields.

Special acknowledgements to our in-house research team:

- Franca Quarneti: research
- Natalia Kesselman: copy editing
- Mariana Venini: copy editing

References

1 Montero, L., Ballesteros-Vivas, D., Gonzalez-Barrios, A. F., & Sánchez-Camargo, A. D. P. (2023). Hemp seeds: Nutritional value, associated bioactivities and the potential food applications in the Colombian context. *Frontiers in Nutrition*, 9, 1039180. doi: 10.3389/fnut.2022.1039180

2 Agricultural Research Service (ARS), United States Department of Agriculture (USDA). Industrial hemp production: Plant characteristics and cultivation overview. https://www.ars.usda.gov/oc/utm/exploring-the-myriad-possibilities-of-hemp/

3 National Institute of Food and Agriculture (NIFA). https://www.nifa.usda.gov/industrial-hemp

4 Shoemaker, J. V. (1899). The therapeutic value of Cannabis indica. Texas. *Medical News*, 8(10), 477–88.

5 Kynett, H. (Ed.). (1895). Cannabis Indica. *Medical and Surgical Reporter (New York)*, 72(1), 569.

6 Abel, L. (1980). *Marihuana: The First Twelve Thousand Years*. New York, NY: Springer. https://doi.org/10.1007/978-1-4899-2189-5

7 Ibid.

8 NORML. (n.d.). Racial disparity in marijuana arrests. https://norml.org/marijuana/fact-sheets/racial-disparity-in-marijuana-arrests/

9 Gunadi, C. & Shi, Y. (2022). Cannabis decriminalization and racial disparity in arrests for cannabis possession. *Social Science & Medicine*, 293, 114672. doi: 10.1016/j.socscimed.2021.114672

10 Sheehan, B. E., Grucza, R. A., & Plunk, A. D. (2021). Association of racial disparity of cannabis possession arrests among adults and youths with statewide cannabis decriminalization and legalization. *JAMA Health Forum*, 2(10), e213435. doi: 10.1001/jamahealthforum.2021.3435

11 Anders, J. (1990). *Beyond Counterculture: The Community of Mateel*. Pullman, WA: Washington State University Press.

12 Miller, C. (2018). Where there's smoke: The environmental science, public policy, and politics of marijuana. Lawrence, KS, University Press of Kansas.

13 Mosher, C. J. & Akins, S. (2007). *Drugs and Drug Policy: The Control of Consciousness Alteration*. Thousand Oaks, CA: Sage Publications, Inc. https://doi.org/10.4135/9781452225806

14 ACLU. (2020, April 16). *A Tale of Two Countries: Racially Targeted Arrests in the Era of Marijuana Reform*. https://www.aclu.org/publications/tale-two-countries-racially-targeted-arrests-era-marijuana-reform

15   https://norml.org/marijuana/fact-sheets

16   Quinnipiac University. (2017, April 20). U.S. voter support for mari-juana hits new high. *Quinnipiac University Poll*. https://poll.qu.edu/Poll-Release-Legacy?releaseid=2453

17   Goode, E. (1997). *Between Politics and Reason: The Drug Legalization Debate*. New York, NY: St. Martin's Press.

18   Anguelov, N. & MacCarthy, M. P. (2018). *From Criminalizing to Decriminalizing Marijuana*. Lanham, MD: Lexington Books.

19   Brienen, M. E. & Rosen, J. D. (2015). *New Approaches to Drug Policies*. New York, NY: Palgrave Macmillan.

20   Cerino, P., Buonerba, C., Cannazza, G., D'Auria, J., Ottoni, E., Fulgione, A., Di Stasio, A., Pierri, B., & Gallo, A. (2021). A review of hemp as food and nutritional supplement. *Cannabis and Cannabinoid Research*, 6(1), 19–27. doi: 10.1089/can.2020.0001

21   Tripathi, A. & Kumar, R. (2022). Industrial hemp for sustainable agri-culture: A critical evaluation from global and Indian perspectives. In D.C. Agrawal, R. Kumar, & M. Dhanasekaran (Eds.), *Cannabis/Hemp for Sustainable Agriculture and Materials* (pp. 29–57). Springer, Singapore. doi: 10.1007/978-981-16-8778-5_2

22   Russo, E. B. (2016). Clinical endocannabinoid deficiency reconsidered: Current research supports the theory in migraine, fibromyalgia, irritable bowel syndrome, and other treatment-resistant syndromes. *Cannabis and Cannabinoid Research*, 1(1), 154–165. https://doi.org.10.1089/can.2016.0009

23   Sebastian, S. V., John, X., Dong, X., Trostle, C., Pham, H., Joshi, M. V., Jessup, R. W., Burow, M. D., & Provin, T. L. (2023). Hemp agron-omy: Current advances, questions, challenges, and opportunities. *Agronomy*, 13(2), 475. doi: 10.3390/agronomy13020475

24   Russo, E. B. (2016). Clinical endocannabinoid deficiency reconsid-ered: Current research supports the theory in migraine, fibromyalgia, irritable bowel, and other treatment-resistant syndromes. *Cannabis and Cannabinoid Research*, 1(1), 154–65. doi: 10.1089/can.2016.0009

25   ACLU. (2020, April 16). *A Tale of Two Countries: Racially Targeted Arrests in the Era of Marijuana Reform*. https://www.aclu.org/publications/tale-two-countries-racially-targeted-arrests-era-marijuana-reform

26   Grinspoon, P. (2016). *Free refills: A doctor confronts his addiction*. New York, NY: Hachette Books.

27   Jobs Report 2022 (2022, February 23). Legal cannabis now supports 428,059 American jobs. *Leafly*. https://www.leafly.com/news/industry/cannabis-jobs-report

28   Quinnipiac University. (2017, April 20). U.S. voter support for mari-juana hits new high. *Quinnipiac University Poll*. https://poll.qu.edu/Poll-Release-Legacy?releaseid=2453

29 Witters, D. (2022). Four in 10 Americans cut spending to cover health-care costs. Washington, D.C.: Gallup Inc. https://news.gallup.com/poll/395126/four-americans-cut-spending-cover-healthcare-costs.aspx

30 Gallup Inc. (2021). West Health-Gallup 2021 Healthcare in America Report. Washington, D.C.: Gallup Organization. https://www.gallup.com/analytics/357932/healthcare-in-america-2021

31 Centers for Disease Control and Prevention. (2023, April 13). *Chronic Pain Among Adults – United States, 2019–2021*. Centers for Disease Control and Prevention. https://www.cdc.gov/mmwr/volumes/72/wr/mm7215a1.htm

32 Hill, K. P., et al. (2017). Cannabis and pain: A clinical review. *Cannabis Cannabinoid Res*, May 1; 2(1), 96–104. doi: 10.1089/can.2017.0017. PMID: 28861509; PMCID: PMC5549367.

33 Webb, C. W. & Webb, S. M. (2014). Therapeutic benefits of cannabis: A patient survey. *Hawaii J Med Public Health*, Apr; 73(4), 109–11. PMID: 24765558; PMCID: PMC3998228.

34 Sharma, R. (2014). *Pursuit of gut happiness: A scientific and simple guide to use probiotics to achieve optimal gut health*. Raams Consulting LLC.

35 Christensen, C., et al. (2022). Clinical research evidence supporting administration and dosing recommendations of medicinal cannabis as analgesic in cancer patients. *J Clin Med*, Dec. 30; 12(1), 307. doi: 10.3390/jcm12010307. PMID: 36615107; PMCID: PMC9821014.

36 McMahon, A. N., et al. (2023). Perceived effectiveness of medical can-nabis among adults with chronic pain: Findings from interview data in a three-month pilot study. *Cannabis*, July 5; 6(2), 62–75. doi: 10.26828/cannabis/2023/000149. PMID: 37484052; PMCID: PMC10361798.

37 Boehnke, K. F., et al. (2020). High-frequency medical cannabis use is associated with worse pain among individuals with chronic pain. *The Journal of Pain*, 21(5–6), 570–81, ISSN 1526-5900. doi: 10.1016/j.jpain.2019.09.006.

38 Carlini, B. H., et al. (2017). Medicinal cannabis: a survey Among health care providers in Washington State. *American Journal of Hospice and Palliative Medicine®*, 34(1), 85–91. doi: 10.1177/1049909115604669

39 Sagy, I. et al. (2018). Ethical issues in medical cannabis use. *European Journal of Internal Medicine*, 49, 20–22, ISSN 0953-6205. doi: 10.1016/j.ejim.2018.01.016

40 Luque, J. S., et al. (2021). Mixed methods study of the potential therapeutic benefits from medical cannabis for patients in Florida. *Complementary Therapies in Medicine*, 57, 102669, ISSN 0965-2299. doi: 10.1016/j.ctim.2021.102669

41 World Health Organization. (2022, February 3). *Cancer*. World Health Organization. https://www.who.int/news-room/fact-sheets/detail/cancer

42 American Cancer Society. (2024). (rep.). *2024 Cancer Facts and Figures* (pp. 1–9). Atlanta, GA.

43   Guzmán, M. (2018). Cannabis for the management of cancer symptoms: THC Version 2.0? *Cannabis Cannabinoid Res*, May 1; 3(1), 117–19. doi: 10.1089/can.2018.0009. PMID: 29789813; PMCID: PMC5961457.

44   Smith, L. A., Azariah, F., Lavender, V. T. C., Stoner, N. S., & Bettiol, S. (2015). Cannabinoids for nausea and vomiting in adults with cancer receiving chemotherapy. *Cochrane Database of Systematic Reviews*, Issue 11. Art. No.: CD009464. doi: 10.1002/14651858.CD009464.pub2

45   Tomko, A. M., et al. (2020). Anti-cancer potential of cannabinoids, terpenes, and flavonoids present in cannabis. *Cancers* (Basel). July 21; 12(7), 1985. doi: 10.3390/cancers12071985. PMID: 32708138; PMCID: PMC7409346.

46   Moreno, E., et al. (2020). The interplay between cancer biology and the endocannabinoid system: Significance for cancer risk, prognosis and response to treatment. *Cancers* (Basel). Nov. 5; 12(11), 3275. doi: 10.3390/cancers12113275. PMID: 33167409; PMCID: PMC7694406.

47   Salamat, J. M., et al. (2022). Interplay between the cannabinoid system and microRNAs in cancer, *ACS Omega* (12), 9995–1000. doi: 10.1021/acsomega.2c00635

48   Tomko, A. M., et al. (2020). Anti-cancer potential of cannabinoids, terpenes, and flavonoids present in cannabis. *Cancers* (Basel), July 21; 12(7), 1985. doi: 10.3390/cancers12071985. PMID: 32708138; PMCID: PMC7409346.

49   Abrams, D. I., (2022). Cannabis, cannabinoids and cannabis-based medicines in cancer care. *Integr Cancer Ther,* Jan–Dec; 21: 15347354221081772. doi: 10.1177/15347354221081772. PMID: 35225051; PMCID: PMC8882944.

50   Häuser, W., Welsch, P., Radbruch, L., Fisher, E., Bell, R.F., & Moore R. A. (2023). Cannabis-based medicines and medical cannabis for adults with cancer pain. *Cochrane Database Syst Rev*, June 5; 6(6), CD014915. doi: 10.1002/14651858.CD014915.pub2. PMID: 37283486; PMCID: PMC10241005.

51   Todaro, B (2012). Cannabinoids in the treatment of chemotherapy-induced nausea and vomiting. *Journal of the National Comprehensive Cancer Network*, 10(4), 487–492. https://doi.org.10.6004/jnccn.2012.0048

52   Braun, I. M., et al. (2024). Cannabis and cannabinoids in adults with cancer: ASCO Guideline Q&A. *JCO Oncology Practice* 0, OP.23.00775. doi: 10.1200/OP.23.00775

53   García-Morales, L., et al. (2023). CBD inhibits in vivo development of human breast cancer tumors. *Int J Mol Sci*, Aug 26; 24(17), 13235. doi: 10.3390/ijms241713235. PMID: 37686042; PMCID: PMC10488207.

54   World Health Organization. (2007, February 27). Neurological disorders affect millions globally: WHO report. World Health Organization. https://www.who.int/news/item/27-02-2007-neurological-disorders-affect-millions-globally-who-report

55 World Health Organization. (2024, March 14). Over 1 in 3 people affected by neurological conditions, the leading cause of illness and disability worldwide. World Health Organization. https://www.who.int/news/item/14-03-2024-over-1-in-3-people-affected-by-neurological-conditions--the-leading-cause-of-illness-and-disability-worldwide

56 Simon, M. & Lipman, M. D. (2020, April 9). Charlotte Figi, the girl who inspired a CBD movement, has died at age 13. CNN. https://www.cnn.com/2020/04/08/health/charlotte-figi-cbd-marijuana-dies/index.html

57 Lattanzi, S., et al. (2018). Efficacy and safety of cannabidiol in epilepsy: A systematic review and meta-analysis. *Drugs*. Nov; 78(17): 1791–1804. doi: 10.1007/s40265-018-0992-5. PMID: 30390221.

58 Haddad, F., Dokmak, G., & Karaman, R. (2022). The efficacy of cannabis on multiple sclerosis-related symptoms. *Life* (Basel), 12(5), 682. https://doi.org/10.3390/life12050682

59 Singh, K., Bhushan, B., Chanchal, D. K., Sharma, S. K., Rani, K., Yadav, M. K., Porwal, P., Kumar, S., Sharma, A., Virmani, T., & Kumar, G., & Noman, A. A. (2023). Emerging therapeutic potential of cannabidiol (CBD) in neurological disorders: A comprehensive review. *Behavioural Neurology*, 2023, 8825358. https://doi.org/10.1155/2023/8825358

60 Hidding, U., Mainka, T., & Buhmann, C. (2024). Therapeutic use of medical cannabis in neurological diseases: A clinical update. *Journal of Neural Transmission*, 131(February), 117–126. https://doi.org/10.1007/s00702-023-02719-1

61 Bhunia, S., Kolishetti, N., Yndart Arias, A., Vashist, A., & Nair, M. (2022). Cannabidiol for neurodegenerative disorders: A comprehensive review. *Frontiers in Pharmacology*, 13, 989717. https://doi.org/10.3389/fphar.2022.989717

62 Singh, K., et al. (2023). Emerging therapeutic potential of cannabidiol (cbd) in neurological disorders: A comprehensive review. *Behav Neurol*, Oct 12, 8825358. doi: 10.1155/2023/8825358. PMID: 37868743; PMCID: PMC10586905.

63 Hidding, U., et al. (2024). Therapeutic use of medical *Cannabis* in neurological diseases: a clinical update. *J Neural Transm*, 131, 117–26. doi: 10.1007/s00702-023-02719-1

64 Bhunia, S., et al. (2022). Cannabidiol for neurodegenerative disorders: A comprehensive review. *Front Pharmacol*, Oct 25; 13, 989717. doi: 10.3389/fphar.2022.989717. PMID: 36386183; PMCID: PMC9640911.

65 Balash, Y., et al. (2017). Medical cannabis in Parkinson disease: Real-life patients' experience. *Clinical Neuropharmacology*, 40(6), 268–72. doi: 10.1097/WNF.0000000000000246

66 Aladeen, T., et al. (2023). Medical cannabis in the treatment of Parkinson's disease. *Clinical Neuropharmacology*, 46(3), 98–104. doi: 10.1097/WNF.0000000000000550

67   Campos, R. M. P., et al. (2021). Cannabinoid therapeutics in chronic neuropathic pain: From animal research to human treatment. *Front Physiol*, Nov. 30; 12, 785176. doi: 10.3389/fphys.2021.785176. PMID: 34916962; PMCID: PMC8669747.

68   Treves, N., et al. (2021). Efficacy and safety of medical cannabinoids in children: A systematic review and meta-analysis. *Sci Rep*, 11, 23462. doi: 10.1038/s41598-021-02770-6

69   Bourke, J. A., et al. (2019). Using cannabis for pain management after spinal cord injury: A qualitative study. *Spinal Cord Ser Cases*, Oct. 8; 5, 82. doi: 10.1038/s41394-019-0227-3. PMID: 31632740; PMCID: PMC6786415.

70   Haleem, & R. Wright, R. (2020). A scoping review on clinical trials of pain reduction with cannabis administration in adults. *J Clin Med Res*, Jun; 12(6), 344–51. doi: 10.14740/jocmr4210. Epub 2020 Jun 4. PMID: 32587650; PMCID: PMC7295551.

71   de Carvalho Reis, R., et al. (2020). Efficacy and adverse event profile of cannabidiol and medicinal cannabis for treatment-resistant epilepsy: Systematic review and meta-analysis, *Epilepsy & Behavior*, 102, 106635, ISSN 1525-5050. doi: 10.1016/j.yebeh.2019.106635

72   Sarris, J., et al. (2020). Medicinal cannabis for psychiatric disorders: A clinically-focused systematic review. *BMC Psychiatry*, 20, 24. doi: 10.1186/s12888-019-2409-8

73   National Academies of Sciences, Engineering, and Medicine; Health and Medicine Division (2017). Board on population health and public health practice; *Committee on the Health Effects of Marijuana: An evidence review and research agenda. The Health Effects of Cannabis and Cannabinoids: The Current State of Evidence and Recommendations for Research*. Washington (D.C.): National Academies Press (US); Jan 12. 4, Therapeutic Effects of Cannabis and Cannabinoids

74   Cuttler, C., Spradlin, A., & McLaughlin, R.J. (2018). A naturalistic examination of the perceived effects of cannabis on negative affect. *J Affect Disord*, Aug 1; 235, 198–205. doi: 10.1016/j.jad.2018.04.054. Epub 2018 Apr 6. PMID: 29656267.

75   LaFrance, E. M., et al. (2020). Short and long-term effects of cannabis on symptoms of post-traumatic stress disorder. *Journal of Affective Disorders*, 274, 298–304. doi: 10.1016/j.jad.2020.05.132. ISSN 0165-0327.

76   O'Donnell, J., Hughes, T., & Innes, S. (2020, January 31). Is marijuana linked to psychosis, schizophrenia? It's contentious, but doctors, Feds say yes. USA Today. https://www.usatoday.com/story/news/nation/2019/12/15/weed-psychosis-high-thc-cause-suicide-schizophrenia/4168315002/

77   World Health Organization. (2023, September 27). Anxiety disorders. World Health Organization. https://www.who.int/news-room/fact-sheets/detail/anxiety-disorders

78 U.S. Department of Health and Human Services. (n.d.). Any anxiety disorder. National Institute of Mental Health. https://www.nimh. nih.gov/health/statistics/any-anxiety-disorder

79 Anxiety and Depression Association of America, ADAA. (n.d.). Facts & Statistics: Anxiety and Depression Association of America, ADAA. *Facts & Statistics.* https://adaa.org/understanding-anxiety/facts-statistics

80 Phan, K. L., Angstadt, M., Golden, J., Onyewuenyi, I., Popovska, A., & de Wit, H. (2008). Cannabinoid modulation of amygdala reactivity to social signals of threat in humans. *J Neurosci,* Mar, 5; 28(10), 2313–9. doi: 10.1523/JNEUROSCI.5603-07.2008. PMID: 18322078; PMCID: PMC2657360.

81 University of Oxford. (2014, July 16). How cannabis causes paranoia. https://www.ox.ac.uk/news/2014-07-16-how-cannabis-causes-paranoia

82 Stoner, S. A. (2017). *Effects of Marijuana on Mental Health: Anxiety Disorders.* Alcohol & Drug Abuse Institute, University of Washington, June http://adai.uw.edu/pubs/pdf/2017mjanxiety.pdf

83 World Health Organization. (2023a, March 13). Depressive disorder (depression). https://who.int/news-room/fact-sheets/detail/depression

84 U.S. Department of Health and Human Services. (2023, July). Major depression. National Institute of Mental Health. https://www.nimh. nih.gov/health/statistics/major-depression

85 Depression and Bipolar Support Alliance. (2019, July 12). Depression statistics. https://www.dbsalliance.org/education/depression/statistics/

86 Sorkhou, M., Dent, E. L., & George, T.P. (2024). Cannabis use and mood disorders: A systematic review. *Frontiers in Public Health,* 12. https://doi.org/10.3389/fpubh.2024.1346207

87 Cuttler, C., et al. (2018). A naturalistic examination of the perceived effects of cannabis on negative affect. *Journal of Affective Disorders,* 235, 198–205. doi: 10.1016/j.jad.2018.04.054, ISSN 0165-0327

88

89 Stoner, S. A. (2017). *Effects of Marijuana on Mental Health: Anxiety Disorders.* Alcohol & Drug Abuse Institute, University of Washington, June. https://adai.uw.edu/pubs/pdf/2017mjdepression.pdf

90 Feingold, D. & Weinstein, A. (2021) Cannabis and depression. *Adv Exp Med Biol,* 1264, 67–80. doi: 10.1007/978-3-030-57369-0_5. PMID: 33332004

91 Langlois, C., Potvin, S., Khullar, A., & Tourjman, S.V. (2021). Down and high: Reflections regarding depression and cannabis. *Front Psychiatry,* May 14; 12, 625158. doi: 10.3389/fpsyt.2021.625158. PMID: 34054594; PMCID: PMC8160288.

92 Veterans Administration. (2018, September 13). How common is PTSD in adults? PTSD: National Center for PTSD. https://www.ptsd. va.gov/understand/common/common_adults.asp

93   https://www.sleephealth.org/sleep-health/the-state-of-sleepheath-in-america/

94   Orsolini, L., et al. (2019). Use of medicinal cannabis and synthetic cannabinoids in post-traumatic stress disorder (PTSD): A systematic review. *Medicina* (Kaunas). Aug 23; 55(9), 525. doi: 10.3390/medicina55090525. PMID: 31450833; PMCID: PMC6780141.

95   Black, N., Stockings, E., Campbell, G., Tran, L. T., Zagic, D., Hall, W. D., ... & Degenhardt, L. (2019). Cannabinoids for the treatment of mental disorders and symptoms of mental disorders: A systematic review and meta-analysis. *The Lancet Psychiatry*, 6(12), 995–1010.

96   Walsh, J. et al. (2021). Treating insomnia symptoms with medicinal cannabis: A randomized, crossover trial of the efficacy of a cannabinoid medicine compared with placebo. *Sleep*, 44(11); November, zsab149. doi: 10.1093/sleep/zsab149

97   Ibid.

98   Lavender, I., et al. (2022). Cannabinol (CBN; 30 and 300 mg) effects on sleep and next-day function in insomnia disorder ('CUPID' study): Protocol for a randomised, double-blind, placebo-controlled, cross-over, three-arm, proof-of-concept trial. *BMJ Open*, Aug. 23; 13(8), e071148. doi: 10.1136/bmjopen-2022-071148. PMID: 37612115; PMCID: PMC10450062.

99   Centers for Disease Control and Prevention. (2022, April 13). What is inflammatory bowel disease (IBD)? Inflammatory bowel disease (IBD). https://www.cdc.gov/ibd/what-is-IBD.htm

100   Professional, C. C. medical. (2021, May 3). Inflammatory Bowel Disease (overview). Cleveland Clinic. https://my.clevelandclinic.org/health/diseases/15587-inflammatory-bowel-disease-overview

101   Mayo Foundation for Medical Education and Research. (2022, September 16). Ulcerative colitis. Mayo Clinic. https://www.mayoclinic.org/diseases-conditions/ulcerative-colitis/diagnosis-treatment/drc-20353331

102   Swaminath, A., et al. (2019). The role of cannabis in the management of inflammatory bowel disease: A review of clinical, scientific, and regulatory information, commissioned by the Crohn's and Colitis Foundation. *Inflammatory Bowel Diseases*, 25(3), March, 427–435. doi: 10.1093/ibd/izy319

103   Ambrose, T., et al. (2019). Cannabis, cannabinoids, and the endocannabinoid system—is there therapeutic potential for Inflammatory Bowel Disease? *Journal of Crohn's and Colitis*, 13(4), April, 525–35. doi: 10.1093/ecco-jcc/jjy185

104   Doeve, B. H., et al. (2021). A systematic review with meta-analysis of the efficacy of cannabis and cannabinoids for Inflammatory Bowel Disease: What can we learn from randomized and nonrandomized studies? *Journal of Clinical Gastroenterology*, 55(9), 798–809, October. doi: 10.1097/MCG.0000000000001393

105 Starrenburg, F. (2019, June 19). IBD patients feel a lot better after being treated with cannabis. Bedrocan. https://bedrocan.com/dr-timna-naftali-ibd-patients-feel-a-lot-better-after-being-treated-with-cannabis/

106 U.S. Department of Health and Human Services. (2024, May 28). Cannabis (marijuana) Drugfacts. National Institutes of Health. https://nida.nih.gov/publications/drugfacts/cannabis-marijuana

107 National Center for Complementary and Integrative Health (NCCIH). (n.d.). Cannabis (Marijuana) and cannabinoids: What you need to know. U.S. Department of Health and Human Services, National Institutes of Health. https://www.nccih.nih.gov/health/cannabis-marijuana-and-cannabinoids-what-you-need-to-know

108 Corroon, J. (2021). Cannabinol and sleep: Separating fact from fiction. *Cannabis and Cannabinoid Research*, 6(5), 366–71. doi: 10.1089/can.2021.0006

109 Morales, P., Hurst, D. P., & Reggio, P. H. (2017). Molecular targets of the phytocannabinoids: A complex picture. *Progress in the Chemistry of Organic Natural Products*, 103, 103–31. doi: 10.1007/978-3-319-45541-9_4

110 Hergenrather, J. Y., Aviram, J., Vysotski, Y., Campisi-Pinto, S., Lewitus, G. M., & Meiri, D. (2020). Cannabinoid and terpenoid doses are associated with adult ADHD status of medical cannabis patients. *Rambam Maimonides Medical Journal*, 11(1), e0001. doi: 10.5041/RMMJ.10384

111 Almeida, C. F., Teixeira, N., Correia-da-Silva, G., & Amaral, C. (2021). Cannabinoids in breast cancer: Differential susceptibility according to subtype. *Molecules*, 27(1), 156. doi:10.3390/molecules27010156

112 Kaul, M., Zee, P. C., & Sahni, A. S. (2021). Effects of cannabinoids on sleep and their therapeutic potential for sleep disorders. *Neurotherapeutics*, 18(1), 217–27. doi: 10.1007/s13311-021-01013-w

113 Riedel, G., Fadda, P., McKillop-Smith, S., Pertwee, R. G., Platt, B., & Robinson, L. (2009). Synthetic and plant-derived cannabinoid receptor antagonists show hypophagic properties in fasted and non-fasted mice. *British Journal of Pharmacology*, 156(7), 1154–66. doi: 10.1111/j.1476-5381.2008.00107.x

114 Wargent, E. T., Zaibi, M. S., Silvestri, C., Hislop, D. C., Stocker, C. J., Stott, C. G., Guy, G. W., Duncan, M., Di Marzo, V., & Cawthorne, M. A. (2013). The cannabinoid Δ9-tetrahydrocannabivarin (THCV) ameliorates insulin sensitivity in two mouse models of obesity. *Nutrition & Diabetes*, 3(5), e68. doi: 10.1038/nutd.2013.9

115 Jadoon, K. A., Ratcliffe, S. H., Barrett, D. A., Thomas, E. L., Stott, C., Bell, J. D., O'Sullivan, S. E., & Tan, G. D. (2016). Efficacy and safety of cannabidiol and tetrahydrocannabivarin on glycemic and lipid parameters in patients with type 2 diabetes: A randomized, double-blind, placebo-controlled, parallel group pilot study. *Diabetes Care*, 39(10), 1777–86. doi: 10.2337/dc16-0650

116   Maione, S., Piscitelli, F., Gatta, L., Vita, D., De Petrocellis, L., Palazzo, E., de Novellis, V., and Di Marzo, V. (2011). Non-psychoactive cannabinoids modulate the descending pathway of antinociception in anaesthetized rats through several mechanisms of action. *British Journal of Pharmacology*, 162, 584–96. doi: 10.1111/j.1476-5381.2010.01063.x

117   Udoh, M., Santiago, M., Devenish, S., McGregor, I. S., & Connor, M. (2019). Cannabichromene is a cannabinoid CB2 receptor agonist. *British Journal of Pharmacology*, 176(23), 4537–47. doi: 10.1111/bph.14815

118   Nakajima, J., Nakae, D., & Yasukawa, K. (2013), Effects of synthetic cannabinoids. *J Pharm Pharmacol*, 65, 1223–30. doi: 10.1111/jphp.12082

119   Ligresti, A., Schiano Moriello, A., Starowicz, K., Matias, I., Pisanti, S., De Petrocellis, L., Laezza, C., Portella, G., Bifulco, M., & Di Marzo, V. (2006). Antitumor activity of plant cannabinoids with emphasis on the effect of cannabidiol on human breast carcinoma. *Journal of Pharmacology and Experimental Therapeutics*, 318(3), 1375–87. doi: 10.1124/jpet.106.105247

120   Oláh, A., Markovics, A., Szabó-Papp, J., Szabó, P. T., Stott, C., Zouboulis, C. C., & Bíró, T. (2016). Differential effectiveness of selected non-psychotropic phytocannabinoids on human sebocyte functions implicates their introduction in dry/seborrhoeic skin and acne treatment. *Experimental Dermatology*, 25(9), 701–7. doi: 10.1111/exd.13042

121   El-Alfy, A. T., Ivey, K., Robinson, K., Ahmed, S., Radwan, M., Slade, D., Khan, I., ElSohly, M., & Ross, S. (2010). Antidepressant-like effect of delta9-tetrahydrocannabinol and other cannabinoids isolated from Cannabis sativa L. *Pharmacology Biochemistry and Behavior*, 95(4), 434–42. doi: 10.1016/j.pbb.2010.03.004

122   DeLong, G. T., Wolf, C. E., Poklis, A., & Lichtman, A. H. (2010). Pharmacological evaluation of the natural constituent of Cannabis Sativa, Cannabichromene and its modulation by Δ9-Tetrahydrocannabinol. *Drug and Alcohol Dependence*, 112(1–2), 126–33. doi: 10.1016/j.drugalcdep.2010.05.019

123   Mosher, C. J., & Akins, S. (2019). *In the Weeds: Demonization, Legalization, and the Evolution of U.S. Marijuana Policy*. Philadelphia: Temple University Press.

124   Tate, K., Taylor, J. L., & Sawyer, M. Q. (Eds.). (2013). *Something's in the Air: Race, Crime, and the Legalization of Marijuana* (1st ed.). New York, NY: Routledge, https://doi.org/10.4324/9780203758380

125   MacCoun, R. J. & Reuter, P. (2001). *Drug War Heresies: Learning from other Vices, Times, and Places*. Cambridge University Press. doi: Cambridge, UK: Cambridge University Press, https://doi.org/10.1017CBO9780511754272

126   Brienen, M. E. & Rosen, J. D. (2015). *New Approaches to Drug Policies*. New York, NY: Palgrave Macmillan.

Interviewed expert consultants

Donald Abrams, MD investigates the clinical benefits of medical cannabis, especially in cancer treatment and advocates for its use as a complementary therapy.
Integrative Oncologist, UCSF Osher Center for Integrative Health
Professor, Department of Medicine

Hemant Kumar Bid, PhD, MS teaches how medical cannabis can be used to treat illnesses from a neuroscience and biochemical perspective.
Assistant Professor, Morehouse School of Medicine
Adjunct Instructor, Saint Louis University School for Professional Studies

Sandra Carrillo, MD advocates for evidence-based education in cannabis in the medical community.
Medical Director, Medicann IPS Medical Cannabis Clinic

Duclas Charles, PharmD is a cannabis expert who is recognized for his ethical considerations in prescribing cannabis.
Pharmacy Manager, Curaleaf
Founder, Black Health Connect

Patricia Frye, MD is exceptionally experienced in guiding pediatric, adult, and geriatric patients through adding medical cannabis to their therapeutic regiment as a primary or adjunct therapy.
Affiliate Associate Professor, University of Maryland School of Pharmacy

Peter Grinspoon, MD is a TedX speaker, author, and physician renowned for his advocacy and educational efforts in medical cannabis.
Primary Care Physician, Massachusetts General Hospital
Instructor, Harvard Medical School

Mara Gordon specializes in developing cannabis treatment protocols for patients with serious illnesses, focusing on data-driven, patient-specific treatment plans.
Co-Founder, Aunt Zelda

Mikhail Kogan, MD focuses on integrative geriatrics and cannabis science.
Medical Director, George Washington University Center for Integrative Medicine
Board Advisor, Doctors for Cannabis Regulation

Paloma Lehfeldt, MD, MA has conducted studies on the use of minor cannabinoids in treating generalized anxiety disorder and advocates for cannabis resource opportunities.
Senior Director of Scientific Communications, Elevation Capital

Chanda Macias, PhD, MBA is a cell biologist who focuses on cannabis research and education, particularly its impact in healthcare and symptom management.
Chairwoman of the Board of Managers and CEO, Women Grow
CEO, National Holistic

Marion McNabb, DrPH, MPH advocates for cannabis research and education.
Senior Director of Research and Learning, United Way of Massachusetts Bay
President, Cannabis Center of Excellence

Marcelo Morante, MD specializes in cannabis for health and neuroscience, various aspects of cannabis use in medical treatments, including the importance of selecting the appropriate delivery method and precise dosing.
Coordinator, Programa Nacional de los usos medicinales del Cannabis
MSAL Argentina

Cheri Sacks, RN, CDCES focuses on integrating digital health technologies with cannabis treatment plans.
Founder and Certified Cannabis Nurse Consultant, Chronic Health Wisdom

Rajiv Sharma researches the endocannabinoid system and its implications in inflammation and cancer.

Monica Werkheiser, PharmD specializes in the treatment of neurological and neurodegenerative diseases.
Head of Operations, Canna Remedies

Genester Wilson-King, MD, FACOG is a nationally recognized speaker on cannabis and wellness who presents on cannabis in obstetrics, gynecology, and women's health.
Founder and Medical Director, Victory Rejuvenation Center

Quoted expert consultants

Jocelyn Elders, MD is the former Surgeon General of the United States and pioneering advocate for drug policy reform.

Manuel Guzmán, PhD is a leading figure in the study of cannabinoids' effects on cancer, neurodegenerative diseases, and metabolic disorders.
Professor of Biochemistry and Molecular Biology, Complutense University of Madrid
Member, Spanish Royal Academy of Pharmacy

Paola Massi emphasizes the potential of cannabinoids as complementary therapies in oncology, and aims to develop effective and targeted cancer treatments.

Timna Naftali, MD is known for her pioneering clinical research on the therapeutic effects of cannabis in managing symptoms and improving the quality of life for patients with Crohn's disease and ulcerative colitis.
Senior lecturer, Sackler School of Medicine, Tel Aviv University

Index

Join the Sheldon Press community today, sign up for our newsletter!

- Select a **FREE eBook** or extract to read upon joining

- Keep up with our latest publishing and exciting author news

- Be the first to hear about book prize draws, free extracts, and upcoming author events

Simply scan the QR code below or head to www.sheldonpress.co.uk/newsletter to sign up.